CONTENTS

diagnosis, identify the patients' problems, encourage patients to help themselves, support patients). Knowledge of PVFS. Patient's role. Other supportive treatment (pain killers, antidepressants, sleeping tablets, anti-fungal measures, vitamins and minerals, detoxification, other measures, conclusion). Summary.

ABOUT THE AUTHOR

Dr Darrel Ho-Yen was born in Guyana, South America, but finished his schooling in London. After a year's Voluntary Service Overseas in the Caribbean, he went to medical school at Dundee University. He completed his training at the Regional Virus Laboratory, Ruchill Hospital, Glasgow. He is now Consultant Microbiologist at Raigmore Hospital, Inverness; Director of the Scottish Toxoplasma Reference Laboratory; and Honorary Clinical Senior Lecturer at Aberdeen University.

Dr Ho-Yen has had extensive experience in managing and counselling patients with Post Viral Fatigue Syndrome and the first edition of this book (1985) was the first book on this subject. The second edition was published in 1987. He is also a co-author of the Oxford University Press textbook **"Diseases of Infection"** (1987 and 1993).

His experience on the needs of patients with chronic illnesses prompted him to write **"Unwind! Understand and control life be better!!"** in 1991. He was also joint editor of **"Human Toxoplasmosis,"** published by Oxford University Press in 1992. Dr Ho-Yen has published numerous scientific papers and articles for medical practitioners and the general public.

PREFACE TO THIRD EDITION

The first edition of this book was the first book on PVFS/ME published. Since then, there has been an avalanche of books on the subject, but only a few have reached a second edition. Similarly, there are many more scientific articles published on PVFS/ME, but again I have been selective in my use of references.

I have been very grateful to the many patients who have been generous enough to comment on the aspects of my book that they found most helpful. Over the years, I have spoken to very many groups of patients throughout Britain. At these talks, many have felt that my pictorial slides were very useful. **Thus, in this edition I have included many of the slides that I use to illustrate my talks.**

This edition has a revised lay-out and more than 60% new material. **The type setting has been designed to be read by individuals able to concentrate for only a short time.** This has meant that there is some repetition so that each chapter can be read independently. **I have received many comments which lead me to believe that this book has a useful purpose in motivating patients, and helping them to adopt a plan for recovery.**

I am very grateful to Mrs Audrey Grant who kindly produced some of the figures. Mr Alan McGinley was responsible for most of the figures in this book and he has shown great understanding and skill in coping with my demands. I am also indebted to Mr John McGhie who has been particularly considerate. Ms Diane Drummond of Words & Images has also been very helpful in the preparation of this book. Lastly, Miss Lorna Wycherley has had the most difficult job of preparing this manuscript for publication through its many drafts. She has shown great insight, understanding, humour and stamina in this task.

8

PREFACE TO THE SECOND EDITION

The first edition of this book was printed in April, 1985. It was in response to numerous requests from patients and doctors for information on the Post Viral Fatigue Syndrome. **I had found that patients needed much support and that hours could be spent on the telephone (at great cost) or in consultation.** At these times I often found myself repeating what I had said before, so it seemed a logical step to write down my approach and opinions. I hoped that this would allow a patient to read a particularly relevant section several times.

I am grateful for the many helpful comments I have received from numerous readers of the first edition. These have prompted me to write several new chapters (on the history of the illness, employment, alternative medicine and self-help groups) and to remove the chapter on Herpes, Hepatitis and AIDS. I had included this latter chapter in the first edition as herpes, hepatitis and AIDS were viral infections which required patients to adopt a different lifestyle and to have a detailed understanding of their illness.

Since this book was first printed, there have been several other books and numerous articles published on the Post Viral Fatigue Syndrome. All such publications are not quoted in this book. I have been selective in quoting published work. **My objective was to formulate a rational approach to the illness, taking into account the available information.** This book is different in that it emphasises what the patient and doctor should do to best cope with the illness. More than 40% of the book has been rewritten. It is hoped that the book will be used as a manual for a change in lifestyle and as a means of support at time of relapse.

Lastly, I am very grateful for the help and support given by Jen, Gregory and Colan during this venture. I am also indebted to Dr V A Spence for his helpful comments on the manuscript, and Miss Edith H Simpson for secretarial help.

DARREL HO-YEN 1987.

CHAPTER ONE

INTRODUCTION

The whole family was sitting down to dinner. As the meal had been late on the table, all of the family were hungry and busy eating. Suddenly, young Gregory announced that he had dived from the one metre diving board and had been congratulated on his perfect entry into the water. There was no immediate response as all the family continued eating. Then, the youngest son, Colan, remarked:

"So what, Gregory? You said that you did that at last week's swimming lesson".

"Yes" said Gregory, thinking as fast as he could "But actually, last week I was pushed".

This book is written for those who are prepared to dive. It is not for those who want to be pushed. Those who are prepared to be active and do are the ones who will be most helped. As Robert Burns stated, "Let us do or die".

VIRAL-LIKE INFECTIONS

The word **"virus"** is derived from the Latin word meaning

"venom" or "poison". In medicine, the word virus is used to describe a very small particle which usually cannot be seen with an ordinary microscope. The study of the behaviour of such particles is called "virology". **However, viral infections can sometimes have a profound effect on human behaviour, both physical and mental (either directly or indirectly).** In many cases, the derivation of virology should probably be entirely different. It may be more appropriate to suggest a derivation from the Latin "vir" (a man) and "logos" (study), thus virology would then be "the study of man".

Everyone has an average 2-7 viral infections every year and these diseases cause over half of the absenteeism from work. The vast majority of people recover from viral infections within a couple of days, or at the most some weeks (Figure 1). **In the few who do not recover, and who develop Post Viral Fatigue Syndrome (PVFS),** the outlook can be bleak. Illness can continue over years, or even decades, and a wide spectrum of complaints can occur. Often, one complaint will linger for months only to be followed with another. Good health appears to be unattainable. **Many patients become depressed and contemplation of suicide is not uncommon.**

Most patients react to their situation by regaling their doctors, family and friends with their complaints. Initially, there is sympathy, but most of the population (including many doctors) do not have any experience of PVFS. **Slowly, the goodwill of those around patients is exhausted, and patients become isolated.** Their demands of their doctor increase. The doctor can respond by referring patients to other doctors and hospitals. Finally, there is the psychiatric referral, with the condolence of both relatives and friends. Patients are the only ones who believe in their own sanity, but even they

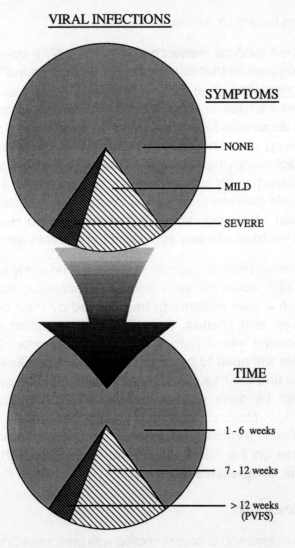

VIRAL INFECTIONS

SYMPTOMS

— NONE

— MILD

— SEVERE

TIME

— 1 - 6 weeks

— 7 - 12 weeks

— > 12 weeks
  (PVFS)

RECOVERY

Figure 1   Viral infections and recovery
Almost all of the population have viral infections, and most infections produce
no symptoms. In those with symptoms, recovery in the majority occurs in 1-6
weeks. A few patients take more than 12 weeks to recover and many of these
will have PVFS.

begin to have their doubts.

Recent medical research shows that PVFS does exist. The suggestion that this illness is "all in the mind" is just not acceptable. Over the last five years, there has been a massive increase in knowledge of this illness. Some of the recent discoveries have been due to the application of modern technology, others have been a result of workers in other areas of medicine applying their expertise to PVFS. Much of this new information has not been extensively communicated, and thus lay people (and many doctors) are not aware of its existence. **One can say unequivocably that there is no reason to doubt the truth of many complaints in patients with PVFS.**

Currently, there are no cures for PVFS. The newly acquired information about the syndrome is, nevertheless, extremely useful. **It allows patients to be believed by their doctors, relatives and friends.** Further, this information can be incorporated into a plan for patients to recover. **Simply, patients will need to become involved in their illness and start to find their own answers to problems.** The ways that this can be done will be discussed and perhaps more important, factors that make the illness worse will be highlighted. **Avoidance of such factors reduces many stresses on the mind and the body, thereby enhancing gradual, progressive recovery.**

TERMINOLOGY

One manifestation of acute infection with presumed Coxsackie virus (described later) is called Bornholm disease. Another name for this disease is epidemic myalgia, as the title of the monograph describing an early outbreak was : "Epidemic myalgia : Bornholm disease". Thus, these two terms are used for a type of acute Coxsackie infection. There has been difficulty in finding an acceptable term to describe the chronic illness. Several names have been used (Table 1).

Table 1   Common names for the illness

Epidemic Neuromyasthenia
Iceland disease (1948-9)
Royal Free Disease (1955-8)
Benign myalgic encephalomyelitis
Myalgic encephalomyelitis (ME)
Chronic Fatigue Syndrome
Post Viral Fatigue Syndrome

Epidemic neuromyasthenia was mainly used in America. **Iceland disease** and **Royal Free disease** were terms used after notable outbreaks in these two places. However, for a worldwide illness association with a particular place is not ideal. **Benign myalgic encephalomyelitis** has been used, however, the word "benign" is only appropriate in that there is not a high mortality. As some patients may have the illness for decades, I do not think benign is appropriate.

Another suggestion has been **epidemic myalgic encephalomyelitis** as this describes the occasional epidemic (large groups of patients affected at the same time) form of the disease. However, most cases are probably sporadic (ie occur in ones and twos as opposed to whole groups), so epidemic is inappropriate. The term **myalgic encephalomyelitis** alone would be more acceptable, and certainly this term with its abbreviation "ME" has been generally used. One criticism of this term is that many patients do not have "myalgia" (muscle pain). In America, the description **Chronic Fatigue Syndrome** has been advocated. This definition requires the exclusion of some 50 conditions and it is possibly less useful. For many patients the illness starts after a viral- like infection, and thus the description **Post Viral Fatigue Syndrome** (PVFS) may be more reasonable. It may well be that PVFS is a less severe form of myalgic encephalomyelitis. It is also possible that a similar clinical picture to PVFS may be occasionally produced by chemicals or other toxins.

I like the term PVFS as it describes the most common clinical condition and it is an easily understood description. The vast majority of patients remember an initiating viral infection and most patients have previously been well, but one needs to remember the limitations in the use of PVFS.

Many have criticised the use of the word "viral " in PVFS as similar illnesses may be caused by infectious agents that are not viruses (such as *Toxoplasma gondii,* or *Borrelia burgdorferi* which causes Lyme disease). However, with PVFS, the "viral" does not imply that all patients have a virus which causes the illness. **Instead, "viral" implies that most patients have a viral-like illness with fever and malaise at the onset.**

THE DOCTOR'S ROLE

The doctor's role in the management of patients with PVFS is critical (Figure 2). He has the responsibility of making a diagnosis, providing information for patients and in motivating them to help themselves. **As the illness is likely to last for some years, the doctor will also have to exclude other causes of further symptoms in the patient.** All of this will take a considerable amount of time, however, it is likely to result in a relationship of mutual trust and respect.

For myself, I can say that a professional relationship can change to one of true friendship. The words of George Washington, the First President of the United States, in a letter

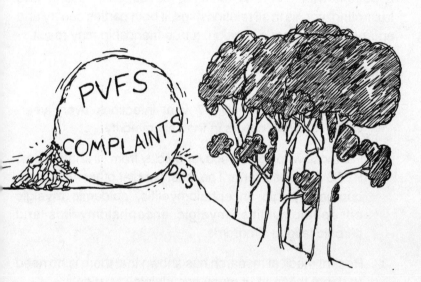

Figure 2   The major obstacle
Most patients see the medical profession as their major obstacle. In the past this was true, but there has been a gradual change in the attitudes of the medical profession. In some areas of Britain as many as 71% of general practitioners accept the existence of PVFS.

of 1783 are as true now as they were then :

"True friendship is a plant of slow growth and must undergo and withstand the shocks of adversity before it is entitled to the appellation."

Loosely interpreted, the relationship between a doctor and a patient with PVFS is likely to be difficult, testing and frustrating; yet, as in all relationships, if both parties can try and appreciate the other's position, a true friendship may result.

SUMMARY

1. Everyone usually has 2-7 viral infections every year. Quick recovery occurs in the vast majority.

2. For those who do not recover quickly from viral infections, PVFS is the best term. The most popular other names are benign myalgic encephalomyelitis, epidemic myalgic encephalomyelitis, myalgic encephalomyelitis and chronic fatigue syndrome.

3. Recent medical research has shown that there is no need to doubt the truth of many complaints of patients.

4. The "viral" in PVFS is not meant to suggest that all patients have viruses as the cause of their illness. Instead "virus" refers to the fact that the majority of patients remember a viral-like illness with pyrexia and malaise at the onset of their illness.

5. The doctor has to diagnose the illness, provide patients with information and motivate them.

6. The doctor and patient need to develop a relationship of trust and understanding.

CHAPTER TWO
THE PROBLEM

The scene was idyllic : a sunny day with mother and young son looking at some newly-hatched chickens. The mother was content with life and remarked to her son :

"Look at these young chicks. Isn't nature wonderful? And how do you think these chicks are smart enough to get out of their shells?" Her young son was eager to run off and play football, his immediate answer was :

"Well Mum, they wouldn't have the problem of getting out of their shells if they didn't get in there in the first place".

WHOSE PROBLEM?

In the past, many doctors looked upon PVFS as a problem which their patients had, and which the patients could have avoided. However, is it reasonable to say that a chicken would not have the problem of getting out of the egg if it was never in the egg? Of course, it is not reasonable! This is not a question of choice it is more one of destiny. Fortunately, circumstances are changing and perhaps the insight of Karl Marx (1818-1883) can be now applied to PVFS : **"Mankind**

19

always sets itself only such problems as it can solve".

The last decade has seen a greater acceptance of PVFS, and perhaps now the conditions are right for researchers to start to find answers in PVFS. **Hopefully, doctors will see PVFS as principally a medical problem rather than one of their patients.**

It is not uncommon to hear : **"I have never felt well since I had the flu a year ago".** Flu (influenza), the common cold and many other viral infections can produce similar symptoms, such as headaches, running noses, coughs, chills and sore eyes. Usually these symptoms clear in a few days or at the most in a few weeks, and then the patient returns to good health.**However, more and more cases are being detected where there is not a quick return to good health.** In these patients, months or years after the acute illness, there are still debilitating symptoms of excessive tiredness and poor recovery after minor activity or stress. In addition, many of these patients have other complaints such as dizziness, difficulty seeing, tremors and pains in different parts of the body. **Why does this happen? And what should these patients do?**

How common are these patients in the general population? **A detailed study in the north of Scotland has shown that doctors found PVFS in 1.3 per 1000 of their patients (Figure 3).** In this study, 71% of doctors accepted the existence of PVFS. This is a particularly high acceptance rate for Britain, but it means that the figure of 1.3/1000 of the population is probably an under-estimate. I estimate that in Britain as a whole about 40% of the medical profession accept the existence of PVFS. There is still a lot to be done in educating doctors.

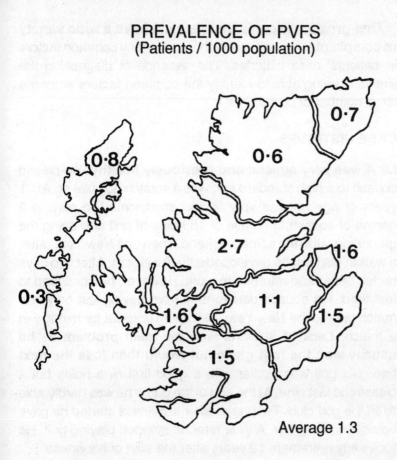

PREVALENCE OF PVFS
(Patients / 1000 population)

0·7

0·8

0·6

2·7

1·6

0·3

1·6

1·1

1·5

1·6

1·5

Average 1.3

Figure 3   Prevalence of PVFS in the North Scotland
There is more illness in areas of greater population. The prevalence varies
between 0.3 to 2.7 per 1000 of the population. For the whole area, 1.3/1000
of the population were affected.
(Ho-Yen D O and McNamara I, British Journal of General Practice,
1991;41:324-326).

21

One great problem is that patients have a wide variety of complaints. Nevertheless, there are many common factors in patients' case histories. The essence of diagnosing the illness is being able to identify the common factors among a large number of complaints.

CASE HISTORIES

Mr A was very athletic and previously healthy. He played squash to a high standard and was a scratch golf player. At 31 years of age he was very fit and accustomed to playing 3 games of squash, 3 games of 18 holes of golf and doing the gardening, all in the same weekend. Then one New Year, after a walk in the hills, he developed a flu-like illness. After two days he felt better and returned to work. However, he continued to feel tired. His squash deteriorated from having lost only one match prior to the New Year, to it being unusual for him to win a match. **Lack of stamina was the main problem as he usually won the first game but would then lose the next two.** His golf was similar with a good first nine holes but a disastrous last nine. At the end of the game he was hardly able to lift the golf club. Two years after the illness started he gave up squash altogther. A year later he stopped playing golf. He took early retirement 12 years after the start of his illness.

Although women and men have an equal chance of developing the illness, it appears that women are more likely to become chronic sufferers. The reasons for this are unknown. Some researchers have suggested that the preponderance of women indicates that PVFS is a hysterical illness. However, the almost equal numbers of men and women affected at the onset of the disease is against such an interpretation.

Mrs B was a 30 year-old, energetic, social worker who

skied and was a good squash player. She developed a "3-day flu" in January one year after which she has never felt well. In the first few months after the illness started, her principal complaint was excessive tiredness. She needed to sleep a lot and could feel tired even after a good night's sleep. **Over the first year, she stopped playing sport and her social life was considerably reduced as she was always tired in the evening.** But the worst was not yet over. In the second year, she developed a rhinitis which resulted in her nose being blocked all day and running all night. Despite numerous tablets and a sinus wash-out, there was no improvement, but instead her nasal secretions produced a cough and breathlessness at night. Later that year, she was admitted to hospital with asthma. By the end of the year, it was felt that she was allergic to dairy products, and she had had further surgery to her nose. At the end of nine years, she still feels exhausted most of the time and her nose still runs.

All ages can be affected by PVFS (Figure 4). Master C was a 9 year-old boy who experienced severe tiredness after a flu-like illness. Over the next year he was an intermittent attender at school and was suspected of having school phobia. However, the education psychologist felt that the boy had an organic illness and a detailed examination of his history showed that he had previously enjoyed school and his activities. With proper management, he slowly returned to good health. **The outlook is much better in younger people. Nevertheless, all ages can show dramatic improvement.**

Whereas most patients become very frustrated with their illness after a few months, the length of time that the illness could last is quite impressive. Mrs D has had pain and fatigue on walking for 15 years. This is in addition to other symptoms which have meant that she has consulted many

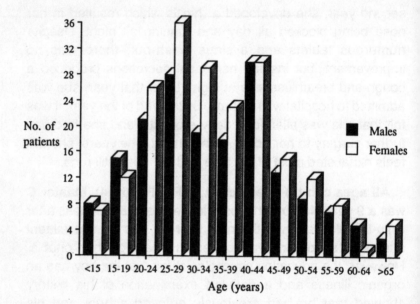

Figure 4   Age distribution of patients
All ages are affected. There is a double peak at 25-29 years and 40-44 years
in both sexes. In this study the sex incidence was almost equal (204F : 177
=1.2F : 1.0M).
(Ho-Yen D O, Scottish Medical Journal, 1988;33:368-9)

doctors in many hospitals. **Mr E** has not been well for 29 years. Apart from being easily tired, he remembers a marked inability to concentrate after the start of the original illness. Over the years as he has got older, **with each minor illness he seemed to develop some more symptoms.** However, there is some consolation in that his tiredness is less worrying now that he is retired than when he was forty.

Common to almost all patients is tiredness and exhaustion after minimal exercise. In most, this produces a need for rest and sleep often accompanied by the frustration of : "All I can do is sleep". **Yet, some patients such as Miss F are unable to sleep properly.** She is excessively tired, goes to bed and sleeps for 3-4 hours, but then awakes. She then spends the rest of the night tossing and turning. Her mind wanders, her muscles twitch and move on their own accord. She gets up, goes to the toilet, has a cup of tea, but still is unable to sleep on returning to bed. Similarly, rest is not easy for **Mrs G who gets intense pain and burning in her muscles after exertion.** The pain is so intense that she needs strong analgesics to dull the pain. She cries herself to sleep when the pain is particularly bad.

Although fatigue can be a very worrying symptom, at least it is a normal sensation and experienced by everyone. **Some of the more unusual symptoms that can occur after viral infections are much more disturbing. Miss H** suffered from shooting pains at the top of her head and in her spine several times a day. **Miss I** has periods when she is unable to say what she is thinking, and when she can speak, she may forget huge parts of the previous conversation. **Miss J** suffered from dizziness which is made worse by travelling in a car or on a bus. This is so bad that even a short journey results in her being totally disorientated and lost. She now walks everywhere.

For many patients, the family is the most important unit. The family, with other members being normal and healthy, is able to offer physical help and moral support. A common statement is : "If it were not for the family, I would have given up a long time ago".

Fortunately, PVFS does not usually affect the whole family. **Yet, for Mr and Mrs K, they have the unusual distinction of both being affected.** Worse still, their 14 year-old son also has PVFS. At the moment, this just appears to be a particularly unlucky combination of circumstances. **Whole families are only rarely affected, although it is not uncommon to have more than one member of the family with PVFS.**

PATIENT GROUPS

There is now much more information available on the groups of patients that develop PVFS (Table 2).

Table 2   Patient groups affected by PVFS
(Ho-Yen D O, McNamara I. British Journal of General Practice, 1991; 41:324-326)

Teachers and students	22%
Retired	16%
Housewives	13%
Service industries	11%
Secretarial/clerical staff	9%
Skilled workers	9%
Unskilled workers	8%
Hospital workers	7%
Professional workers	5%

Most patients are in groups most exposed to infection. Among the unskilled workers, some were illiterate and so could

26

not be influenced by magazine articles. Not surprisingly with so much ill health, many of these patients exhaust the patience of their doctor, extended family and friends. When this happens the illness can be further complicated by depression, anxiety, paranoia and the contemplation of suicide.

Many patients are hoping for a "cure" from the medical profession. Yet, to most doctors viral infections usually do not last longer than a few months, and hospital laboratories are principally designed to detect viral infections in the first few months of the illness. **Thus, patients feeling unwell years after a viral infection are not catered for by the traditional medical service.** Help for these patients lies in their own ability to understand their illness and to adopt attitudes that change their lifestyle, thus increasing their chances of recovery.

SUMMARY

1. PVFS is not an uncommon illness, with at least 1.3 per 1000 of the population being affected.

2. In one study, 71% of general practitioners accepted the existence of PVFS. However, for the whole of Britain the figure is probably about 40% of the medical profession.

3. Many patients were previously athletic, very productive individuals and accustomed to good health. The vast majority of patients were previously healthy.

4. Women and men have equal chance of developing the illness, but women may be more likely to become chronic. There is a double peak of PVFS at 25-29 years and 40-44 years.

5. All ages may be affected, but the out-look is much better in younger people. In some patients, illness may last many decades. Occasionally, families are affected.

6. Patients need to understand their illness and change their lifestyle to increase their chances of recovery.

CHAPTER THREE
HISTORY OF PVFS

There is the story of the tourist, Ron, visiting some of the monasteries in Greece. At each monastery, he was met by a dedicated monk and given a learned commentary on the history of the monastery. Touring was hard work and Ron found it difficult to concentrate. He was content to look at the icons and enjoy the soft breeze blowing through the monastery. He was in a dream. He looked forward to the end of the tour which was marked by the monk producing a religious relic, for which generous contributions could be made. As he reached for his wallet, the monk was finishing :

"This is the child's skull of St. Andreas, our patron Saint".

Several days later, at the end of another tour, he was aware of another monk producing a bigger box and commenting :

"This is the skull of St. Andreas, our patron Saint".

Ron, awakened, exclaimed :

'Wait a minute! Two days ago, I was shown a child's skull and I was told that the skull was that of St. Andreas".

"Ah yes", replied the monk "that one must have been of St. Andreas as a child".

For many, the history of PVFS has a similar curiosity. Some have been preoccupied by a first description.

OUTBREAKS

Several authors have stated that the first outbreak was in Los Angeles in 1934. The accepted early outbreaks are as in Table 2. They cover the last 60 years and show a truly worldwide illness.

Table 3   Notable outbreaks of PVFS

Los Angeles   (1934)
Switzerland   (1937-39)
Australia   (1949-51)
New York   (1950)
Middlesex   (1952)
Coventry   (1953)
Athens   (1958)
London   (1970)
West Kilbride   (1980-83)
Stirlingshire   (1983)

I shall summarise important aspects of previous outbreaks. Many areas of the world have been affected, from North America (Los Angeles, 1934; New York, 1950; Washington, 1953; and Florida, 1956) to Europe (Switzerland, 1937; Iceland, 1948; and Athens, 1958) and Australia (1949). **Thus, both temperate and tropical areas have been involved, but most outbreaks have been in tropical countries.** Of note is that Britain has had many outbreaks (London, 1952, 1964 and 1970; Coventry, 1953; Newcastle upon Tyne, 1959; and West Kilbride, 1980). Four of these outbreaks have been in closed communities: three in hospitals (Middlesex Hospital, a Coventry hospital and the Hospital for Sick Children, Great

Ormond Street) and one in a Teacher's Training College. Two of the outbreaks were in general practice and thus both small and large groups, closed and open communities may be affected.

The importance of the sex of the patients has been considered by some to be critical. The hypothesis is that as in some outbreaks women seem to be mainly affected; then, the case for the outbreak being due to hysteria becomes strong, as hysteria is more common in women. Apart from being chauvinistic, this hypothesis does not consider all the available evidence. There are outbreaks that have been confined to army personnel (ultimately "macho"), as in Switzerland in 1937 and 1939.

The most likely explanation of apparent sex difference is that infection spreads more quickly in groups of people : irrespective of the sex of the group, the group becomes infected. **Overall, there are probably more women affected than men, but this difference is not great and certainly not sufficient for "hysteria" to be the explanation of the PVFS.** For each outbreak, there is probably only one virus responsible. However, virological evidence for such an assumption has only been obtained in the Scottish outbreaks in West Kilbride and Balfron. In these cases, the Coxsackie virus was implicated; in the other outbreaks, the diagnosis of PVFS was made clinically and there was no convincing evidence of a viral infection. This is not a criticism, but only a comment that it is very difficult to obtain acceptable virological data. **Thus, patients should not be disillusioned if, in their particular case, there is no evidence of a viral infection.**

One problem with an emphasis on outbreaks is that it can be forgotten that most cases are sporadic. At any one time, there may be 10-20 different viruses circulating in the community. PVFS may be a rare complication of any or all of these viruses. Not all of these viruses can be easily tested for in the laboratory. This is why a diagnosis of a viral infection is often made on the clinical picture. **There is a temptation for patients to blame their doctor for not having the wit to request the correct test.** If there is to be any blame, it is best put at the door of current, medical, virological and immunological investigations. **These investigations are not adequate to answer the questions being asked.**

WHY ME?

Why me? Or, why ME (myalgic encephalomyelitis, Post Viral Fatigue Syndrome)? These are frequently asked questions by patients and their relatives. **Many patients believe that the answer to these questions is in medical research.** I would like to emphasise that "research" literally means "to search again". As with all searching it helps if you know what you are looking for and where to look (Figure 5), but sadly this information is not available with PVFS. **Thus, medical research offers only long-term solutions. Patients should therefore find more immediate solutions to their problems.**

I do not believe that the earliest outbreak of PVFS was in 1934. **I believe that PVFS has existed for as long as there have been viral infections - from the very start of man's existence.** Obviously, the limitations of early descriptions depend on documentation. Most cases of PVFS are sporadic (i.e. do not occur in outbreaks) and cases occuring in ones and twos are less likely to be documented. This is an important consideration. Doctors in the past, with fewer journals and fewer doctors, were unlikely to record individual cases or small outbreaks. To be documented, an outbreak had to be large.

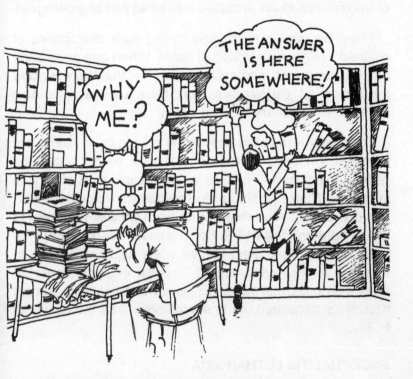

Figure 5   Why ME?
Why me? Or why ME (ME/PVFS). Many people believe that the answer to this question is in research. However, it helps if you know what you are looking for and where to look. The answer may be here somewhere, but would we recognize it if we saw it? Research provides only long-term solutions.

Further, centuries ago the expectation of good health was much less. People expected to be capable of doing less as they got older. People died earlier. Thus, there were fewer cases and individuals accepted their lot as part of growing old.

Therefore, one is more likely to find early descriptions of outbreaks rather than individual cases. **When one goes back into the historical, medical records, I feel that there is good evidence of outbreaks that take us back to the seventeenth century.**

The usefulness of this exercise in delving back into history is limited. Yet, there is no doubt that some cannot accept the general hypothesis - PVFS is a rare complication of all viral infections. **Where you have viral epidemics (especially with some viruses), you are going to have greater numbers (a minor epidemic) of PVFS.** For those who cannot accept the general hypothesis, there can be some help and support in evidence of previous outbreaks. This evidence can reassure these individuals that the disease is not new. It is this argument which has stimulated me to search again into the history of PVFS.

ENCEPHALITIS LETHARGICA

What is this? Why is it not heard of now? These are good questions. **Even to the layman, lethargy and somnolence coupled with disease of the brain (encephalitis lethargica) has some similarity to PVFS.** In addition, there is evidence that the disease occurred in all age groups, but chiefly in the 20-30 age group; social status and occupation played no part in determining those affected. I believe that encephalitis lethargica was an early description of severe PVFS.

An early account was probably the encephalitis

lethargica outbreak in Copenhagen 1657. Cases of the disease appeared to be related to epidemics of fevers, most likely influenza. After the 1918-1919 pandemic of influenza which killed 20 million people worldwide, a large outbreak of encephalitis lethargica followed. One reason for this is that the influenza strain of the 1918-1919 was probably derived from swine. **This particular variant may be neuropathogenic (i.e. particularly likely to attack the nervous system).** When there was widespread vaccination with swine influenza vaccine in the United States in 1976, there were many cases of Guillain-Barré Syndrome (a nervous illness causing paralysis) complicating vaccination. Today, such cases are not seen as complications as swine influenza has been removed from the vaccine.

There have been no widespread outbreaks of swine influenza since 1918-1919, and coincidently there have been no outbreaks of encephalitis lethargica. As this swine variant of influenza is much more toxic to the nervous system than other variants of influenza, it produced late complications of Parkinson's disease in many who had had encephalitis lethargica. Thus, those with severe illness did not have PVFS or ME as we know it. However, descriptions of those with mild encephalitis lethargica are comparable to descriptions of PVFS.

It is possible to say that encephalitis lethargica encompasses the full spectrum of PVFS/ME. This complication was widespread because the variant of influenza infected so many people. When millions are infected, it is not surprising that thousands may develop a PVFS-like illness.

ARBOVIRAL ENCEPHALITIS

Many arboviruses (viruses that are arthropod- borne i.e. insect transmitted) produce encephalitis. Well-documented complications are fatigability, weakness, drowsiness, inability to concentrate and nervousness. **Some were described as "convalescent-fatigue syndrome".** One epidemic of St. Louis encephalitis in 1933 (Journal of the American Medical Association 1938; 111: 15-17) not only shows many similarities to PVFS, but also is instructive on the aftermath of an epidemic. When asked: "Has health been the same, better or worse since the attack of encephalitis?" Responses showed 42% to be the same, 34% to be worse and 24% to be better. **It is perhaps quite revealing to PVFS patients to know that 24% of people can feel better after a viral infection.**

Other interesting findings of this outbreak were that mainly adults were involved, and many were incapable of working (Chapter Fourteen). Two-thirds of the patients studied were restored to good health with only 7% with total disability. This figure is probably a reasonable indication of the prognosis in PVFS. **Again, the degree of disability can vary with the type of virus, being worse in the winter type as compared with the summer type.**

There are several hundred arboviruses with most in tropical countries. It is likely that the frequency of PVFS as a complication of arboviral infection is dependent on the virus. Probably all such viruses have the potential for rarely causing PVFS, but a few viruses (such as St. Louis encephalitis virus) are frequent causes of the syndrome.

SUMMARY

1. Outbreaks of PVFS have been well documented, but in only a few has a virus been implicated. Descriptions of outbreaks divert attention from the importance that all viruses may rarely cause PVFS and that most cases are sporadic.

2. The questions : Why me? Or why ME/PVFS? are frequently asked. Many patients feel that the answers are in medical research. Sadly, these are long-term answers and patients need to find more immediate solutions to their problems.

3. The full history of PVFS is unknown. It probably dates back to the start of man's existence.

4. Encephalitis lethargica and arboviral encephalitis are good candidates for early descriptions of PVFS.

CHAPTER FOUR
INFECTIONS

Everyone enjoyed laughing at Timothy Dexter. His manners were terrible and his clothes were bizarre. He had left school at eight years and never learnt to spell. But Timothy Dexter had one great gift : he was adept at making money. **It did not matter how ridiculous the project was, if his money was involved, the project was certain to be a financial success.** His rivals complained that he was just lucky, but it was more than luck. Money-making was his destiny.

Timothy Dexter enjoyed other's company although he was always the brunt of their jokes. He listened to his so-called friends. They took advantage of him but he always seemed to triumph. Today, his business ventures would be regarded as the ultimate in lateral thinking. In the eighteenth century, he was an object of ridicule. Most of the laughter was premature. Many who laughed did not care that irrespective of the peculiarity of the venture that the result was always good.

A hoaxer told Dexter that there was a shortage of coal in Newcastle. With his limited education; he did not realise that

Tyneside was one of the largest coal producing areas in the world. He bought shiploads of coal and sent them to Newcastle. The story was quickly spread and for weeks it was the most popular joke. **Yet, when the ships arrived in Newcastle, there was a coal strike. Everyone wanted his coal and he made a massive profit.** His so-called friends persuaded him to send warming pans and woollen mittens to the West Indies. Dexter did not realise that a swim suit is sometimes too warm in this tropical paradise. Again, destiny was with the man. His ship's captain was resourceful and sold the warming pans as giant ladles for the large West Indian molasses industry. The woollen mittens were quickly bought by Asian merchants and re-exported to Siberia. Dexter's entry in his diary was perhaps one of great insight :
"I was very lucky in spekkelation".

Despite buying the grandest house in New England and acquiring the English title of "Lord", Dexter was shunned. **No one visited him; no one invited him to dinner.** His snobbish neighbours probably did not appreciate the nettle of the man. At 50 years, he wrote a book which was to become a great oddity of American literature. Entitled "A Pickle for the Knowing Ones or Plain Truths in a Homespun Dress", it was a sell-out. Although intended to be autobiographical, it was bought for its comedy value. Serious readers had a difficult job as there was little punctuation.

As always, Dexter had a perverse reaction to criticism of his variable writing style. His later editions had an extra page which had nothing on it but punctuation marks. He explained "The Nowing ones complane of my book the first edition had no stops I put in A nuf here and they may pepper and salt it as they please".

Timothy Dexter existed. He was a man who despite

those around him managed to live his own life. If he did not exist, he would have to be invented. This is because the public like to have someone to laugh at. Yet, one important consideration was that Dexter was usually right. To many, somehow this did not matter. **Today, it is the same and people are prepared to laugh at others for no good reasons.**

VIRAL-LIKE INFECTIONS

Infections are much like Dexter, if they did not exist, they would have to be invented. In addition, much that is said about infections is untrue, but somehow it does not matter. PVFS can be produced by many infections, but the vast majority are probably caused by viruses. As stated before, **the viral in PVFS refers to the fact that the vast majority of patients remember a "viral-like" illness at the onset with fever, muscle pain and malaise.** There are many causes of viral-like infections (Figure 6). The most common cause of such illnesses are viruses. However, because viruses are so common and difficult to diagnose, doctors usually do not try to find laboratory evidence of such infection.

VIRAL INFECTIONS

Viruses are very small agents which produce a variety of illnesses. **They are very much smaller than bacteria and are so small that they cannot be seen through a normal microscope.** To get some idea of the size of a virus is difficult. Nevertheless, a useful simile is that an apple is just as much larger than a virus as Mount Everest (the highest mountain in the world, 29,028 feet) is higher than the apple.

There are thousands of viruses. Some infect animals and

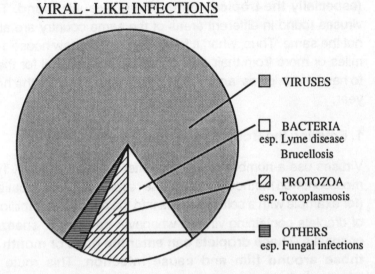

VIRAL - LIKE INFECTIONS

- VIRUSES
- BACTERIA
  esp. Lyme disease
  Brucellosis
- PROTOZOA
  esp. Toxoplasmosis
- OTHERS
  esp. Fungal infections

Figure 6   Viral-like infections
These are produced mainly by viruses, but also by bacteria and protozoa.
Unless specific laboratory investigations are undertaken, it can be difficult to
identify specific causes of such illnesses. The attraction of the name PVFS
is that it describes the early, clinical illness. PVFS does not mean that viruses
are the only cause of the disease.

41

plants and others infect human beings. Common diseases that are produced by viruses are measles, rubella (German measles), mumps, influenza, hepatitis A and B, chickenpox and the common cold. **In different countries of the world (especially the tropics), different viruses are found.** The viruses found in different areas of the same country are also not the same. Thus, when a family moves to a new house 100 miles or more from their old house, it is not unusual for them to have more 'colds' and viral illnesses than usual for the next year.

1. Entering the Body

Viruses use a number of ways to enter the human body. The most common method is through the respiratory tract. A patient (for example with a cold) releases into the atmosphere millions of droplets containing viruses whenever he coughs, sneezes or speaks. **These droplets can enter the nose or mouth of those around him and cause infection.** This route of infection is that used by the common cold and influenza viruses and also those causing childhood diseases, such as mumps, measles and rubella. A susceptible person can become infected by shaking the contaminated hands of a patient with any of these infections, and then touching his own nose or mouth.

Saliva is also a source of infection, especially in respiratory infections. More indirectly, virus can be passed from one person to another, especially through the conjunctivae in the eyes, by sharing towels or even from swimming pools. Contact with infected animals, more so in the tropics, is another source of viral infection.

Another route of infection is the alimentary tract. In certain patients, especially those with hepatitis A, or Coxsackie infections **the virus multiplies in the alimentary tract and passes into the faeces.** In areas with poor sanitation, these infected faeces may contaminate the drinking water and thus cause widespread infection. **Untreated sewage may be discharged into rivers where they can contaminate shellfish, such as oysters.** If these shellfish are eaten raw, they can cause infection. Because of the large amounts of virus that can be excreted in faeces, it is also important that food handlers have high standards of hygiene. If hands are not washed after using the toilet, food may be contaminated and can easily cause infection.

The skin is also an important way by which a virus may enter the body. In patients with cold sores (due to herpes infection), viruses are present in the sores, and thus, contact with these lesions can produce infection. **Penetration of the skin** occurs with bites from bloodsucking insects or animals (for example in the spread of rabies). Drug addicts sharing syringes and needles commonly transmit infection (usually hepatitis B and the HIV/AIDS infection) among themselves.

Although there are many ways for a virus to enter the body, **transmission of viruses from one person to another may not necessarily result in infection.** Infection only occurs if there is enough virus, the patient is susceptible and the virus is able to replicate. **If patients have not had a previous infection with a particular virus, they are susceptible, otherwise they are said to be immune.** Unfortunately, there are hundreds of viruses that can cause the common cold, so it is unlikely that anyone can be totally immune to all colds. Whereas, people usually only have one attack of measles, chickenpox or mumps. Artificial immunity to some viruses may be acquired through vaccines.

2. Viral Replication

Viruses can only replicate (or multiply) within living cells. This is because they do not have the machinery to produce their own offspring. Instead, they hijack a living cell's machinery and utilise it to produce viral offspring. The whole process is complex (Figure 7). The process of viral replication occurs in all viral infections. It demonstrates that infection is a result of a complex series of manoeuvres. **The statement "just a viral infection" is a gross underestimation of the sophistication of viral infections.**

3. Symptoms

Symptoms are what patients complain about when they are ill. The majority of viral infections do not result in any illness and so are called **asymptomatic.** Viruses that regularly produce symptoms are termed **virulent.** There is a period between the virus getting into the body and when the first symptoms appear. During this **incubation period,** the virus is multiplying and spreading to specific parts of the body. **Different viruses attack particular organs** (for example hepatitis A and the liver, or the skin in measles and chickenpox). Characteristic clinical pictures of viruses can allow doctors to diagnose specific diseases.

OTHER INFECTIONS

Other infections may also produce a viral-like illness. (Figure 6). Although bacterial infections are common causes of infection, Lyme disease and brucellosis are the most important in producing PVFS. **Lyme disease** is caused by *Borrelia burgdorferi* and infection is transmitted by a tick bite. Usually there is a characteristic rash (erythema chronicum migrans) at

VIRAL REPLICATION

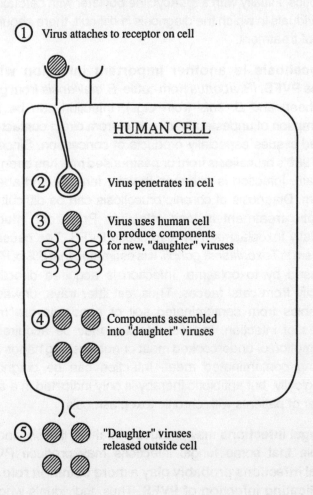

① Virus attaches to receptor on cell

HUMAN CELL

② Virus penetrates in cell

③ Virus uses human cell to produce components for new, "daughter" viruses

④ Components assembled into "daughter" viruses

⑤ "Daughter" viruses released outside cell

Figure 7   Viral replication
This starts with the attachment of the virus to a human cell and finishes with the release of many "daughter" viruses. These are capable of infecting other cells and the whole process may be repeated many times over. It is a sophisticated and complex process.

the site of the bite and joints may be affected. Treatment is with antibiotics, initially with a tetracycline but later with cefotaxime. In individuals in which the diagnosis is difficult, there should be a trial of treatment.

Brucellosis is another important infection which causes PVFS. (*B. abortus* from cattle, *B.melitensis* from goats and sheep and *B. suis* from pigs). Infection can be from consumption of unpasteurised milk, or from direct contact with infected tissues especially products of conception. Since the early 1980's brucellosis from unpasteurised milk has been rare in Britain. Infection is common in vets, farmers and abattoir workers. Diagnosis of chronic brucellosis can be difficult and antibiotic treatment is less effective. Protozoal infection especially toxoplasma may also cause PVFS. The causative organism is *Toxoplasma gondii.* It is estimated that 5% of PVFS is caused by toxoplasma. Infection is acquired directly or indirectly from cats' faeces. Thus, cat litter trays, unwashed vegetables from contaminated soil or sand pits are major sources of infection. Indirect infection may be acquired by consumption of undercooked meat or not washing hands after handling contaminated meat. Infection can be diagnosed serologically, but antibiotic therapy is only indicated in a small number of patients with chronic toxoplasmosis.

Fungal infections may produce a viral-like illness, and it is possible that some fungal infections may produce PVFS. **Fungal infections probably play a more common role as a complicating infection of PVFS.** Thus, individuals who are ill with PVFS may be more susceptible to fungal infections such as *Candida albicans* infection. Treatment of such complicating infection may improve the PVFS but would not cure it.

IMMUNOLOGY

The immune system protects the body against infections. **As any system in the body, it may be normal, less active or too active.** In patients with PVFS, this spectrum of activity can also be found. Some patients complain of developing every infection that is around, and in these patients their immune system may have reduced function. Others complain of never actually developing an infection but feeling as though they are about to have an infection. In these patients, the body's immune system may be activated so that infections do not have time to develop.

The symptoms of PVFS may be produced by two mechanisms : reduced ability of the immune system to deal with infection; or, by the immune system becoming activated after an infection and unable to switch itself off. This latter mechanism is akin to a country prepared for battle, in which all invaders (infections) are rapidly repelled, but the resources of the country are being used up by the army. It is likely that both mechanisms exist at different times of the illness, or in different individuals.

An important group of cells in the body's immune system are the lymphocytes. There are four important sub-populations of lymphocytes : **B lymphocytes** which produce antibodies against specific infections; **T- helper lymphocytes** which help other cells to destroy infectious agents; **T-suppressor lymphocytes** which stop the body's immune response; and **natural killer cells** which are the body's first-line of defence against infections.

In PVFS, the immune response appears to vary in different parts of the world (Table 4). Different causative agents may produce different immune responses. The best explanation of

47

the results in Table 4 is that **in different parts of the world, the major causes of PVFS are different.**

Table 4   Worldwide immune responses in PVFS.

Study	T-h	T-s	NK
America	Raised	Normal	Normal/Reduced
Australia	Reduced	Normal	Normal
Scotland	Normal	Raised	Normal/Raised

The results of the NK cells variations in the Scottish study led the authors to speculate on a series of events (Figure 8).

DIAGNOSIS

Doctors suspect that a virus is causing a patient's symptoms by the type of symptoms. Also, as viruses produce infectious illnesses, the doctor may have seen several other patients with similar symptoms. In the early stages of the illness, the virus can be grown or seen by an electron microscope from samples taken from different parts of the body. In later stages, the virus cannot be grown or easily seen, but changes in the blood may indicate that there is a current infection.

These changes are of two types. First, **there are non-specific changes** which show that the patient has an infection, but there is no indication of the cause of the infection. Secondly, **there are specific changes** indicative of a particular infection. These are usually antibodies which are produced by the body's lymphocytes to help to kill the virus. **Unfortunately, there can be great difficulties in diagnosing viral infections.** Problems often occur in patients who are ill for months or years. Attempts to grow the virus are usually futile because in only a few cases are symptoms due to continuing

SEQUENCE of EVENTS

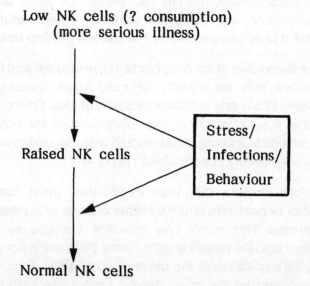

Low NK cells (? consumption)
(more serious illness)

Raised NK cells

Stress/
Infections/
Behaviour

Normal NK cells

Figure 8   NK cell sequence of events
It is postulated that there is an initial low NK cell result (probably because of consumption of NK cells fighting the infection or a serious illness); the body responds by producing a raised NK cell result to combat the infection; finally, the NK cell result returns to normal as the body recovers. Progress to subsequent stages is influenced by stress, infections and behaviour.
(Ho-Yen D O et al. Scandinavian Journal of Infectious Diseases 1991; 23:711-716).

infection. Of the several syndromes that can occur after a viral infection, the PVFS is probably the most common. Here, symptoms are due to the prolonged effects of the infection on the body, especially its immune system. Medical research (British Medical Journal, 1983; 287: 85-8) has shown that immunological abnormalities can persist for years after an acute infection, and **when the immune system returns to normal it is accompanied by the patient getting better.**

The diagnosis of chronic bacterial, protozoal and fungal infections may be equally difficult. Again, investigations may have to be done in specialised laboratories. Often, results are only supportive rather than diagnostic of the condition. Immunological investigations should also be undertaken as these may identify abnormalities (Table 4).

Before doctors diagnose PVFS, they must consider whether or not there could be other causes of the patient's symptoms. This is not only essential, but also serves to reassure both the patient and the doctor that there is not a more easily treated cause of the patient's complaints. Thus, PVFS is diagnosed by the characteristic history, excluding other causes of the patient's symptoms, finding evidence of a viral infection and by demonstrating immunological abnormalities.

SUMMARY

1. In PVFS, the viral refers to "viral-like" illnesses which are usually caused by viruses, but also by bacteria, protozoa and fungi.

2. There are thousands of viruses of animals, plants and man. They can gain entry into the body in many ways, but infection only occurs if there is enough virus, the patient is susceptible and the virus is able to multiply.

3. Multiplication of a virus is a sophisticated, complex process. When sufficient 'daughter' viruses are produced, symptoms occur in a minority of patients. The majority have no symptoms.

4. The immune system is responsible for the body's defenses. In PVFS, symptoms may be produced by a reduced or increased activity of the immune system.

5. There are worldwide differences in T-helper, T-suppressor and natural killer cells which may be related to different infections causing PVFS in different countries.

6. Diagnosing an infection depends on growing the organism or finding evidence of the organism in the blood. Unfortunately, diagnosis of chronic infections is not easy.

CHAPTER FIVE
SYMPTOMS AND DIAGNOSIS

An old, weather-beaten farmer came into the surgery one day to make an appointment for the doctor to see his wife.

"Gladly," said the doctor "Is she ill?" "Well, I'm not exactly sure, doctor" "What is she complaining of?"

"She doesn't really complain, doctor" replied the farmer "But, take yesterday. She got up at 4 o'clock, milked the cows, made breakfast for the family, washed the clothes, cleared the barn, made the month's cheese, cooked lunch, planted the vegetables, weeded the garden, made dinner, did the washing-up and started the sewing. Then, without any warning, at 11 o'clock at night she started saying she felt tired. I think, doctor, that you will have to give her a tonic or something to pick her up".

One person's expectation of good health can be quite different from another person. Thus, some feel that they are ill if they cannot do the work of two normal people. Whilst someone else may describe good health as "having no pain". Good health is therefore open to individual interpretation and expectation.

SYMPTOMS

What a patient complains of (his/her symptoms) is a personal, subjective opinion. It is difficult for other people to fully appreciate the severity of the symptoms. "Agonising pain" for one person may be just "uncomfortable" for another. A description of "a tickling sensation in the arms" was so severe for one patient that it was "torture", whereas another patient described the same sensation as "a wonderful, relaxing feeling".

Symptoms of infection such as fever, malaise muscle pain and tiredness are commonly found either individually or together. **Most such complaints are due to viral infections, but other infections can produce a similar clinical picture.** Any other symptoms that the patient may have influences the doctor to make a diagnosis, for example a scarlet rash is indicative of the bacterial infection of scarlet fever.

Viral infections are complicated as they may be acute, chronic or latent. Acute infections are usually over in a few weeks, and rarely last some months. **Chronic** infections last months or years. **Latent** infections are when the virus remains quiet in the body in between bouts of illness (for example, shingles or cold sores). Symptoms of acute infections are well known : the characteristic rash of chickenpox, measles or rubella; the salivary gland enlargement of mumps; the running nose, cough and fatigue of the common cold or influenza; and the yellow skin (jaundice) of hepatitis A and B.

Less well known is that other viruses are common causes of respiratory tract infection, diarrhoea or infection of the nervous system. **Any part of the body can develop a virus infection,** and the medical literature has evidence of viruses producing symptoms in every system of the body.

Generally, most people recover from a viral infection in a few weeks. The recovery is complete and the patient feels as well as he did before the infection. However, in a small number of cases this does not happen. In these patients, the acute infection lasts longer and then the acute symptoms stop, but there is no return to good health. Instead there is a prolonged period of ill health. This results in a number of characteristic conditions of which the most common is probably PVFS.

The symptoms are usually not due to the acute infection (which has passed), but to the effects of that acute infection on the body. Over the subsequent years, the body will slowly recover, but in the meantime there are things that the patient can do that will produce a better recovery.

COMPLICATIONS OF VIRAL INFECTIONS

After a severe viral infection, in which the patient may be comatosed and admitted to hospital, debilitating symptoms would be usual and even expected. Such complications are usually not seen as a consequence of mild infections, but a minority (those with PVFS) may develop these symptoms.

A much smaller group of people have even more unusual symptoms. These symptoms are individual and may only occur in that patient. For that patient, his complaints are as real as any other, but again, because of the medical profession's limited knowledge, such patients may be treated with disbelief. Obviously, because of the unusual nature of the symptoms, other causes must be considered and excluded before these complaints are attributed to PVFS.

Nevertheless, as every cubic inch of the body has millions of cells, it is not surprising that infection may occasionally

produce individual, bizarre symptoms. To some extent, descriptions of symptoms are a reflection of a patient's use of language. Examples of such descriptions are "inability to sit", "hair falls out and then grows again", "hair changes colour", "hears the national anthem", or "smells apples".

As the illness progresses, symptoms may disappear and new symptoms arise. Thus, patients may initially be particularly worried about muscle pain, but after a few years, headaches may be the major complaint. Similarly, a patient may adjust to tiredness but find it quite difficult to come to terms with difficulty in finding the right words (dysphasia). Generally, the longer the illness progresses, the complications become worse. **This is a great incentive for patients to try and get better soon. Sadly, many patients want to get better but adopt behaviour patterns that makes recovery unlikely.**

POST VIRAL FATIGUE SYNDROME (PVFS)

It is likely that many infections, especially viral infections can cause PVFS, however, it is particularly common after certain infections. Thus, **Epstein-Barr virus** which causes infectious mononucleosis (commonly called glandular fever) is characterised by a sore throat, enlargement of the lymph nodes in the neck, a prolonged fever and malaise with fatigue. It does not occur in outbreaks. A popular description of **infectious mononucleosis** is "the kissing disease", as infection often occurs from transfer of the virus in saliva during a kiss. Fortunately, many develop immunity to the virus during childhood without ever knowing it. **Coxsackie infections** do not usually produce any symptoms, but sometimes a variety of syndromes may develop. Acute infection produces infection of the brain (with headache, vomiting, pain in the eyes when looking at lights, and stiffness of the neck and spine), heart

55

(with severe pains in the left chest) and muscles **(Bornholm disease)**. Bornholm is a Danish island where the disease was first described in 1872. Apparently nearly a quarter of the island's inhabitants developed the illness after attending a wedding feast. One 10 year old boy "suddenly threw himself down on the lawn, screaming" because of the pain in his side. Similar outbreaks **(epidemic myalgia)** have been described all over the world, and in America the disease was called **"devil's grip"** because of the severity of the pain.

Coxsackie infection is spread from faeces of infected persons. **The outlook is good and patients do not die from the disease, although during the illness they may feel that they are about to die.** The acute disease often only lasts a few days, but occasionally persists for a few weeks. In only a very small minority is there persistence of symptoms and development of the PVFS.

From the above, it is apparent that these infections are not new diseases. What is new is the recognition that in a minority of patients, PVFS develops. Nevertheless, some doctors do not accept its existence and may question the truthfulness of the patient. **Many patients with PVFS are unjustly accused of malingering.**

SYMPTOMS OF PVFS

The symptoms of PVFS are many and varied. The most common complaint is fatigue, from which the syndrome derives its name. Other symptoms are best divided into: general, muscular, vascular, neurological, gastrointestinal, cardiac and respiratory. This division is artificial and many symptoms overlap the divisions, for example tiredness is a general symptom but may be related to muscular weakness or neurological anxiety about being tired. Yet, there is some value in looking at the symptoms in the above grouping, especially in patients who have difficulty in explaining what is wrong to friends and neighbours.

Another common complaint is the feeling of ill-health **(malaise)**. This general complaint is usually accompanied by excessive tiredness and exhaustion. **In some patients their inactivity is accompanied by increased sweating, and worse, well-wishers saying that they should rest more as they were sweating.** Explanations by the patient are regarded with disbelief. After all, to the average citizen, one sweats when one is active, anything else is just outside his sphere of understanding.

Muscular problems are again present in the majority of patients. There can be muscle pain, weakness, tremors, twitches, heaviness, cramp, burning and easy fatigue or a persistent feeling of unsteadiness. Some researchers believe that such complaints may be explained by abnormalities in the brain. However, others have described quite extensive disorders of the muscle. **It is possible that there is both muscle and brain dysfunction. Abnormal vascular function is quite common. Cold or very warm hands and feet can be confusing, paradoxical complaints.**An explanation may be related to sex as women often complain of the cold, whereas men more commonly have warm extremities. Nevertheless, it is also not uncommon for patients to change their complaints. Thus patients may complain of great heat and ask for all the windows to be left open and heating turned off in the middle of winter. A few months later these same patients may require four blankets in the middle of summer because of the cold. Such major changes in attitudes can be particularly difficult for spouses. In both sexes, friends may comment that there is loss of colour in the face. **This could be described as "pallor" or even a "grey, mask-like appearance".**

Neurological symptoms are probably the most diverse, and perhaps the most worrying. Headaches may last several weeks and cause the patient much anxiety. Light-headedness, dizziness, sensitivity to temperature, ringing in the ears, blurred vision and sore eyes are common complaints. Difficulty in speaking or finding the right words, poor memory, tingling in the limbs or loss of sensation in different parts of the body are less common. Fears, depression, poor concentration and contemplation of suicide are much more complex symptoms and will be dealt with in a separate chapter (Chapter Seven).

Gastrointestinal symptoms are very common and in many cases may be related to the development of food intolerance or allergy. A feeling of not being hungry (anorexia) can occur on its own or is sometimes related to the patient's frustration with his/her illness. Not surprisingly, in this group weight loss can be a sequel. Diarrhoea can vary between a few extra stools each day to "streaming, almost like water with a horrible smell" which may occur over ten times a day. **Many complain of alternating diarrhoea and constipation.** Vomiting is very rare and must be distinguished from nausea at the sight of food. Pain in the abdomen and a feeling of abdominal distension is common and may be a result of gastrointestinal muscle dysfunction.

Cardiac and respiratory complaints can be a part of the acute illness. When they persist, as part of PVFS, their severity is much reduced. Pains in the chest, awareness of the heart beating **(palpitations)** and difficulty in breathing **(dyspnoea)** are the usual symptoms. Attacks may not be predictable, but in some patients, certain events or certain times of the day precipitate attacks.

TIME TO RECOVERY

The length of time that symptoms persist is a constant source of anxiety for patients, their relatives and their friends. Most people's experience of a viral disease (and in many cases their doctor's experience) is of an acute illness, lasting at most a few weeks. **Whereas this is absolutely true, equally true is that most people's experiences are very limited.** Anyone prepared to read the medical literature would be convinced, because of the numerous descriptions of individual cases and of outbreaks of illness, that the effects of a viral illness can persist for years. It is reasonable to expect to be better tomorrow. It is also reasonable to expect to win the football pools, or to be a national newspaper's millionaire bingo winner. **It is unreasonable to plan your life in the expectation of rapid recovery, or winning a fortune.** Such expectations put a strain on a patient's recovery, and worse when they do not materialise, depression follows. **A superior approach to the problem is to plan a change of lifestyle and a gradual recovery over months or years.** Support from relatives and friends on this basis is much more constructive, and more, such help reinforces any progress that is made.

The vast majority of patients recover within the first year. Of the remainder, most recover within two years. If a patient is ill for a longer time, the chances of recovery progressively decreases. **This is largely because the length of illness is a reflection of a patient's ability to change his/her lifestyle.** The longer that individuals have been trying to do this without success, the less likely are their chances of success. It is similar to passing the driving test. The longer a

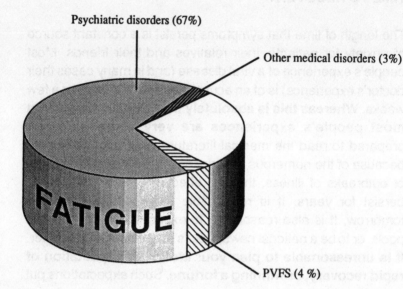

Figure 9 Fatigue

If the complaint of fatigue is considered, the majority of patients (67%) will have a psychiatrical disorder. However, if a strict definition of PVFS is used (Table 5), only about 4% of patients with fatigue will have PVFS. A small number (3%) will have another medical disorder.

person has been trying to pass the test, the chances of success becomes less. **Nevertheless, it is possible for patients to recover even after many decades of illness.** Similarly, Mrs Miriam Hargrave passed her driving test at her 40th attempt after 212 lessons when she was aged 62 years.

Why do people find it so difficult to accept that recovery may take years, and that some people may never totally recover? Everyone would understand gradual improvement after a serious car accident. If there is a diagnosis of advanced cancer, any improvement would be looked upon as a miracle. **Attitudes to viral infections are different because there is nothing to see (unlike the car accident), and people's experiences are limited.** They do not realise that some viral infections can have an effect on the body very similar to cancer.

DIAGNOSIS

Ideally the diagnosis of PVFS should be made by a doctor. **Unfortunately, it is wrong to think that the diagnosis could be made in a patient with just fatigue.** Fatigue can be caused by many conditions. Indeed, fatigue is a common complaint in patients with psychiatric disorders, (Figure 9). This is one of the reasons why some patients with PVFS are believed to have a psychiatric illness.

Table 5   Diagnostic criteria for PVFS
(Ho-Yen DO. British Journal General Practice, 1990); 40:37-39)

Definition

The patient with post-viral fatigue syndrome :
1. has had generalised, relapsing fatigue exacerbated by minor exercise causing disruption of usual daily activities usually (50%) for at least three months.

2. complains of prominent disturbance of concentration and/or short term memory impairment.
3. has no other *obvious,* organic causes for a similar syndrome.

Supporting evidence
(at least four items from sections A, B and C)

A. History

Patient well before illness
An initiating viral illness (clinical description/viral serology)
Myalgia
Gastrointestinal disturbance
Headaches
Depression
Tinnitus
Paraesthesiae
Sleep disturbance
Cardiovascular complaints
Adverse effect of alcohol
Adverse effect of heat

B. Clinical
Lymphadenopathy
Localised muscle tenderness
Pharyngitis

C. Laboratory
Evidence of viral infection
Abnormalities in immune function

It is important that the doctor takes a detailed history and makes a full clinical examination. **Several hundred** conditions may produce a similar illness and it is the doctor's responsibility to exclude any other cause of the patient's complaints.

INVESTIGATIONS

Several initial investigations apply to most patients, and the following are usually normal :

1. Haemoglobin
2. White cell count and differential count
3. Plasma viscosity (or erythrocyte sedimentation rate)
4. Thyroid function tests

In individual patients, it may be appropriate to attempt to identify specific causes of PVFS. A respiratory infection screen and coxsackie neutralisation tests should be done. If tick bites are common, Lyme disease should be excluded. In patients with recurrent sore throats, Epstein-Barr virus infection should be considered. Persisting lymphadenopathy is also a feature of Epstein-Barr virus infection or toxoplasmosis. If facilities are available it can be useful to demonstrate immunological abnormalities (Chapter Four).

Any additional medical condition indicated by the patient's history or clinical examination should be excluded. It is also usual to administor a questionnaire to detect any psychological disorder. The Hospital Anxiety and Depression (HAD) questionnaire (Acta Psychiatr Scand 1983;67:361-370), or a questionnaire for general medical settings (British Medical Journal 1988; 288:897-900) are both useful.

SUMMARY

1. PVFS probably follows any viral infection. It most commonly follows Epstein-Barr virus infection and Coxsackie virus infection (Bornholom disease or epidemic myalgia).

2. Symptoms of PVFS are many and varied. Fatigue is the most common complaint and from which the syndrome gets its name, but any system of the body may be involved.

3. Patients may take years to recover and should plan for gradual recovery rather than an instant cure. Support from relatives and friends on this basis is much more constructive.

4. Diagnosis of PVFS should be made by a doctor. A strict definition of PVFS should be used. If one considers only fatigue the patient is most likely to have a psychiatric disorder.

5. Routine investigations should be performed on all patients. In individual patients, other investigations may be indicated after a detailed history and clinical examination has been performed.

CHAPTER SIX
THE SOLUTION

The "Little People" have always had a fascination for children. In the famous incident of the Cottingley fairy photographs, two young girls claimed to have photographed fairies in July 1917. It later transpired that the girls had used cut-out fairy figures to fake the photographs. However, what is more interesting is that the girls admitted to faking the photographs but still insisted that they had seen the fairies. The reason that they faked the photographs was that adults did not believe their stories.

One can understand children having a vivid imagination, but when an adult recounts a childhood experience it should perhaps be given further consideration. Thus, should the story by Mrs G Herbert in 1928 that she saw a "little wizened man eighteen inches high. It had a little pointed hat, slightly curved at the front, a doublet and little short knicker things," be dismissed? Often the children are not alone when they have witnessed the presence of the Little People. In 1929 a 5 year-old girl and her 8 year-old brother saw a tiny pilot in a plane with a wing-span of 15 inches fly over their garden fence. Whilst 3 girls in Kilkhampton saw a "little man in a tiny red car driving around in circles". More recently, in 1979 4 children (aged 8-10 years) saw about 60 people riding around in little red and white cars.

For patients with PVFS it is important to note a number of characteristics of the Little People. First of all, these accounts show that the Little People are usually driving around, often with mechanised transport. Secondly, the descriptions mention that the Little People were "very happy looking", and that in their presence the children were "awfully happy". I feel that patients with PVFS can greatly benefit from looking at their illness as an invasion of the Little People. **The illness will have catastrophic effects on their lives, but there is also the possibility of much happiness.**

THE CURRENT POSITION

Before one is able to find a solution to problems, it is necessary to have an accurate assessment of the current position. Most patients would describe their current position as "a disaster", "chaos", or "grief and mega-grief". **Whilst these expressions are colourful, and perhaps true, it is better to have an assessment that is factual rather than emotional.** Therefore, "I cannot cope with my job" is more useful than "My life is a disaster". Simply, one can devise a strategy to cope with facts but to deal with an emotional problem may be impossible.

Many patients are very influenced by adverse reports in the media. Such articles and programmes are often interpreted as direct criticism by the patient. This emotional reaction is very difficult to deal with and may even cause a relapse (Figure 10). **This is sad and unnecessary. Patients should recognise that the media frequently gets its facts wrong.** When

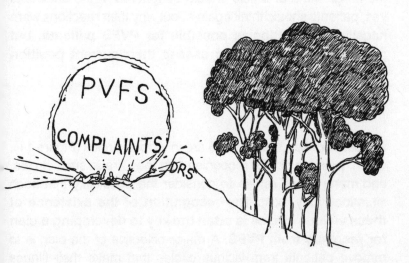

Figure 10   A setback
Adverse reports in the media may be interpreted by patients as direct criticism of themselves. Such reports have been known to cause a relapse. This is an emotional reaction. Patients should recognise that the media frequently gets the facts wrong.

patients see or hear adverse comments, they should not react with anger, horror or disgust. Instead, they should ask the simple question : "Are the facts correct?" If the answer is no, the programme or article should be ignored. If the answer is yes, patients should think again about why their reactions were negative. **A solution is possible for PVFS patients, but patients must first try to assess their current position without too much emotion.**

VICIOUS CIRCLES

Almost all patients with PVFS are in vicious circles (Figure 11). Often, patients do not recognise that they are in such circles, and many would refuse to consider the possibility that such situations may exist. **The recognition of the existence of these vicious circles is often the key to developing a plan for recovery from PVFS.** A major objective of the plan is to remove patients from vicious circles that make their illness worse.

Many patients with PVFS were high achievers before their illness and one of great regrets is the lack of achievements that comes with the illness (Figure 11). The isolation of minimal activity, little money, and no social life is difficult to cope with, especially as many patients were previously "the life and soul" of parties. Close relationships, especially sexual ones, undergo tremendous strain and this matter will be dealt with in greater detail in Chapter Eleven. With most patients, there is a recognition that their current position is one in which they are in vicious circles. **They see no way that they can extricate themselves from these circles. The solution is to adopt the steps for better recovery as described below.**

68

VICIOUS CIRCLES

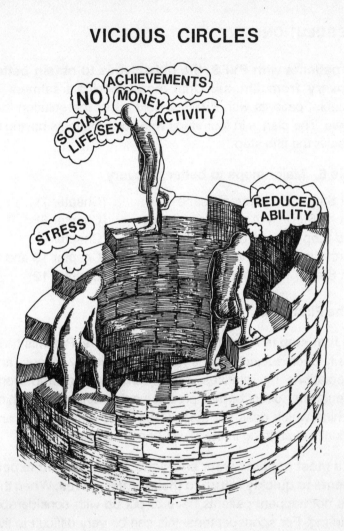

Figure 11 Vicious circles
Patients are in vicious circles. Under-performance in a variety of areas can produce tremendous stress. This stress produces further, reduced performance. The essence of a plan for PVFS patients is for them to get out of vicious circles.

THE SOLUTION

For patients with PVFS, the objective is to obtain better recovery from illness. Until more specific treatment is available, patients with PVFS should adopt the solution that follows. The plan is in four steps with some patients having to consider the fifth step.

Table 6   Major steps to better recovery

First Step :	Remain sane	(Chapter 7)
Second Step :	Acquire knowledge	(Chapter 8)
Third Step :	A daily diary	(Chapter 9)
Fourth Step :	Understand energy	(Chapter 10 and 11)
Fifth Step :	Food and diets	(Chapter 12)

1. The First Step

The first step is for patients to remain sane. Patients have usually been subjected to ill health, disbelief by friends, and expectations by relatives. Many have had to stop work. Patients often describe their predicament as being in a washing machine which does not stop. There is no time to think and gradually everything in their lives becomes disrupted.

As most patients were energetic, those around expect patients to quickly return to their former selves. When this does not happen, patients have to put up with considerable bantering. For sportspersons, this can be very difficult to live with, especially as prior to their illness they probably had identical views. Thus, it is important that patients realise that they are ill even though relatives and friends may not believe them. Equally important, is for patients not to expect instant cures. Too much time and energy is wasted in the pursuit of these miracles. When these do not materialise, there is further disappointment and depression. **The key to maintaining one's sanity is to develop a resistance to social pressures, and to recognise that recovery will take a long time.**

2. The Second Step

The second step involves the patient acquiring knowledge about the illness. With knowledge, the patient can become involved and committed. Patients start to find answers to their problems, rather than leaving it to doctors, friends or luck. Fear of the future is best overcome with knowledge. **Knowing that recovery is gradual should remove the compulsive expectation of overnight cures, and the frustration that develops when spectacular improvement does not occur.**

Knowing that one's illness can be alleviated or made worse by a range of factors, should lead to a more rational ordered lifestyle. **A patient's anger, frustration and bitterness is usually directed against the medical profession.** Instead, this energy could be better used by patients in understanding more about their disease. With this knowledge, patients will begin to find their own answers rather than expect someone else to provide reassurance. **Instead of replying to magazine adverts which do not live up to their claims, patients should direct their efforts at changing their lifestyles.** This change will reduce the severity of symptoms and the frequency of relapses. Further, there will be the realisation that there is an association between what patients do and how they feel. **Most relapses are not random but are a result of the patient's excesses.** In early illness, they occur within hours or days of the excess. Later in the illness, it may take a week to manifest itself. **The second step requires patients to spend much time learning about their illness.**

3. The Third Step

The third step is a daily diary. To be most helpful, a diary should be every day. It need not be more than a few lines and it does not have to be in sentences. The patient should also attempt to be objective. Many patients would say that over a period of years they had become steadily worse. This is very unusual in PVFS. Commonly, there is a very small but gradual improvement with time. Occasionally, a patient may develop different problems, for example chest pain, and these can create the impression that one is getting worse. **With time patients often forget exactly how bad they were, and one way to monitor the slow improvement is to keep a diary.** Information should be detailed so that it can be consulted in the future, for example, if diarrhoea is a problem, the patient's emotional reaction to the diarrhoea ("this is hell on earth", "I'm about to die") is not as useful as a record of how many times a day it occurs.

Although this step is time-consuming and boring, good records are comparable to a good compass. If one were given the task of traversing unfamiliar terrain, it would be virtually impossible without a good compass. For the patient with PVFS, the walk would be further complicated by being at night with a heavy mist. **The compass would ensure that one was going in the right direction until other landmarks became apparent.** Similarly, patients need to be reassured that they are improving (or at least, not getting worse), and good records would indicate that the direction was right. In addition, should there be deterioration, the records could be examined to find a precipitating factor (or, where the patient has made a wrong turning). Records, although tedious, provide definite landmarks and so a few minutes must be made every day to keep a detailed diary.

Even though the diary must be kept daily, the greatest value is seen when the records are examined over a long period. One usually feels little change from day to day, or week to week. Yet, there may be significant change from what one felt, or was capable of doing months or years previously. The more precise the records, the more change can be noted. PVFS is a chronic illness with a slow recovery, at first often in minor details. **Another great asset of the diary is that it is an emotional safety-valve.** One needs to talk (or write) about one's illness, but patients often behave in extremes - either saying too much or nothing. Instead, all of the great details, frustration and anger should be recorded in the diary. This would allow one to be more rational and say something (but not very much) about one's illness socially, after all, it is a major preoccupation!

4. The Fourth Step

The fourth step is to understand energy. This is the most difficult of all of the steps. Over many years, I have realised that patients find comments such as "moderate your activities" or "stay within your energy levels" impossible to understand. There is a language barrier. **Thus, the unique system of thinking of energy in terms of money was evolved, and has helped very many patients** (Chapter Ten). With this system, patients consider themselves in debt; debt is repaid by restricting spending and by gaining more money through sleep and relaxation.

Stress and relationships also use up great energy (Chapter Eleven). Stressful activities such as worrying over a job or arguments with partners can use as much energy as running up a hill. It is only recently it has been realised that patients should also be aware of energy consumption because of stress. Patients can stay in bed all day, but if they have been stressed there is no benefit.

The general public associates exercise with health, and even that one can become healthy through exercise. Most patients with PVFS would agree with this. Indeed, many are former sportsmen and women, and thus remember a time when they exercised and felt better for it. **The fourth step is the realisation that the body has changed and can now only tolerate limited exercise. It is not a matter of getting the muscles fit again.** The muscles behave abnormally when compared to normal muscles. When a battery is run down, one does not make it better by using it, but rather by allowing it to recharge. The muscles of patients with PVFS need time to become normal again. **Excessive exercise makes matters worse.** With the help of the diary, one can demonstrate this for oneself. Initially, the effect is immediate, but later in the illness it is delayed for up to a week (as the muscles have started to approach normality).

It may be difficult for patients to give up sporting activities, but it is important that they do. Recovery depends upon adopting a new lifestyle. The alcoholic cannot make a new start by continuing to drink. Similarly, patients with PVFS must also give up their addiction to exercise. One benefit is that they will have more time to concentrate on getting better.

Another old fear is that too much sleep is bad. Again this relates to healthy individuals. Those with PVFS are not healthy. For these, sleep is the way that the body has of saying that things are not well and that one needs to slow down. **In addition, sleep is a curative process in which the body is attempting to rectify the damage.** With normal individuals, the fitter one is (or the more one exercises) the less sleep one needs. **The opposite is true for patients with PVFS. The**

74

more they exercise the more sleep they will need.

5. The Fifth Step

Whereas the first four steps are applicable to all patients, the fifth step is only important to some. A proportion of patients who find that they are getting worse, despite the measures that have been advocated, should consider this step.

The fifth step involves an understanding of food. Food probably has an effect on patients in many ways. In some patients, abdominal complaints are severe whilst other patients are unaffected. While food allergies are probably uncommon, food intolerance is more recognised. In addition, patients who have been chronically ill usually derive considerable benefits from an understanding of food. **This is much less important in the recently ill.**

DOCTORS AND HOSPITALS

Many patients react with "But what about the doctors? After all, it's their job to make me better". Although this is essentially true, in PVFS there is no effective treatment currently available. Management depends upon maintaining the patient's sanity and attempting to alleviate any symptoms that are present. **The traditional medical approach of treatment with drugs and tablets is doomed to failure. Recovery is best achieved by patients changing their lifestyle to take into account their body's changed capabilities.** The doctor's role is secondary - not to treat PVFS, but to ensure that the patient does not have any other treatable illness. In particular, when new symptoms develop, doctors and hospitals are able to provide reassurance that there is no other cause of the symptoms by the use of traditional, diagnostic methods. **Patients, knowing that PVFS** is responsible can then start to understand their symptoms and modify their behaviour accordingly.

CHANGE IN LIFESTYLE

Better recovery does not mean immediate recovery. There is *only* slow, gradual recovery from PVFS. What can be learnt is that if life is lived in the same way as before the viral illness, recovery will be even slower. **Instead, a change of lifestyle will allow a better and faster recovery,** especially if the change takes into account the different needs of the body after a viral infection. It is hoped that sufficient information will be provided in this book to enable patients to adopt a positive approach to their illness. It is similar but better than having a leg amputated. With one leg patients have to learn a different approach to life's problems, and eventually hardly notice that they have one leg. **For patients with PVFS, they also have to learn a new way of life, but for them eventually things return to normal - their leg regrows!!**

76

SUMMARY

1. Patients are frequently distressed by adverse reports in the media. They should recognise that the media frequently gets its facts wrong.

2. Patients are in many vicious circles which they may refuse to recognise. A recognition of these circles is the key to developing a plan for better recovery.

3. The plan for better recovery involves five major steps. It is not easy and many patients will not have sufficient commitment to make the plan work.

4. Doctors and hospitals are of secondary help - to exclude other treatable illnesses.

5. Better recovery from PVFS is achieved by a change in lifestyle. Involvement in the illness and commitment by the patient are essential for the difficult task of achieving recovery.

6. All patients have to decide if this plan asks too much of them. It is not sufficient to read this book. Patients need to do what is required.

CHAPTER SEVEN
FIRST STEP: REMAIN SANE

There is the story of Wee Ted who entered the tree-felling competition at the Lumberjack World Championships. Ahead of him were tall, massive lumberjacks who were able to cut a tree down in 20 seconds. When Wee Ted's turn came, there was mocking laughter everywhere. Amazingly, he cut his tree down in 10 seconds. The audience was aghast, and one lumberjack said :

"Where did you learn to fell trees like that?"

"The Sahara." Wee Ted replied.

"But there are no trees in the Sahara." quipped another lumberjack.

"Not any more." replied Wee Ted.

Patients with PVFS have to be like Wee Ted and have faith in themselves, even when the available evidence seems to be against them.

They will be surrounded by apparently more able and knowledgeable people. Yet, the truth is what matters. If they know what their problems are and what has caused them, they must believe in themselves. **This is more difficult, but more sensible than taking advice from well-wishers who have no understanding of the problem.** Better recovery from viral infections cannot be achieved unless patients maintain their sanity. This must be done even though they may be surrounded by a society that tests their sanity. **It is helpful to remember that most people have little experience of delayed recovery after a viral illness.**

EMOTIONS

There is the age-old conundrum : what came first, the chicken or the egg? The relationship of emotion and immunity is complex (Lancet, 1985; ii : 133-34). Patients' emotional state may influence the function of their immune system. Reduced levels of IgA immunoglobulins and increased T (helper) cells have been found in individuals under stress. **It is possible that the patients' emotional state may predispose them to a viral infection, and to delayed recovery from that infection.** Some evidence for such a hypothesis has been found in patients with infectious mononucleosis (Psychosomatic Medicine, 1979; 41 : 445-47).

Alternatively, it may be argued that before the illness, patients were well and that it is the illness itself which has produced the emotional abnormalities. Further, the other social and work consequences of the illness may also produce such effects, even if the initial illness does not. Suffice to say, in patients with PVFS, there is usually a history of a viral infection and abnormal emotions. Like the chicken and the egg analogy, we have both and what came first is of academic importance. **The patient with PVFS has to cope with the aftermath of his viral infection and his emotions; what came first is academic.** Nevertheless, the vast majority of PVFS patients do not have a history of great emotional disturbances. Patients find themselves with many emotional problems (Table 7)

Table 7   Emotional problems

	Problem	Frequency
1.	Fatigue	Always
2.	Depression	Common
3.	Anxiety	Common
4.	Paranoia	Rare
5.	Suicide	Very rare

FATIGUE

The most common complaints of patients with PVFS are fatigue (asthenia) or tiredness. Associated complaints are malaise and weakness (lassitude). Malaise is a general feeling of ill-health. Weakness is the patient's perception that the muscles have reduced strength. **Fatigue is a state of tiredness in which the patient lacks energy and is unable to do much.** Obviously fatigue and weakness blend into each other, and sometimes they cannot be separated.

Of patients' complaints, fatigue and weakness are the most frequent and complex. This is not surprising as these symptoms are a description of ill people. More than half the admissions to a general hospital will also have these complaints. However, for many doctors these symptoms may also suggest psychiatric problems, especially if the results of tests are negative. **Thus, many patients with PVFS may at some stage be referred to a psychiatrist.**

As stated previously (Chapter Five), patients with PVFS require more than fatigue before the diagnosis can be made. Indeed, a great mistake of the uninformed is that they tend to assume that patients with PVFS have only fatigue. With strict diagnostic criteria, in patients with fatigue for a long time, only 4% have PVFS (Figure 9); the majority of patients who only complain of fatigue will have a psychiatric disorder. **If these facts were more widely known, many mistakes by the media would be avoided.**

PSYCHIATRIC DISORDERS

Many PVFS patients could develop some of the complaints of psychiatric disorders. The nature of PVFS, the loss of good health, the length of the illness and the lack of quick treatments may all combine to have adverse effects on patients. **Patients should be aware that there are several time bombs : depression, anxiety, paranoia and suicide.** Fortunately, most patients do not develop full-blown psychiatric disorders.

1. Depression

Depression or unhappiness is a common human emotion. It is a normal, healthy reaction to some of life's problems. It is only a medical problem when it is uncontrollable or if there is no obvious cause for the depression. **Thus, for patients with PVFS, it is not abnormal to be occasionally depressed about tiredness and easy fatigue, indeed it is normal and even necessary.** But, if the depression occurs all the time, then, the behaviour is abnormal. The situation is further complicated by the fact that depression itself can cause tiredness and easy fatigue.

2. Anxiety

Anxiety is a feeling of unease, apprehension, uncertainty

and fear. With anxiety, unlike ordinary fear, the unease is out of proportion to the reason for the fear. Thus, patients with PVFS may be anxious about going shopping or being in large crowds. Indeed, in such situations many have panic attacks. **Panic attacks are sudden, short-lived anxiety attacks.** Although this may be difficult to understand, I believe that in PVFS patients that this is a reflection of the increased concentration required for such activities, and the patients' realisation that they may not be able to cope. **Such patients are often able to easily cope with these situations when they start to recover.**

3. Paranoia

Paranoia is the development of feelings of suspicion and wariness of those around. There is a tendency to blame others and gradually delusions develop, with feelings of self-importance and entitlement. Patients with PVFS find it difficult to understand how those around have only a very limited interest in the patient's symptoms, or length of illness. Relatives and friends are quickly bored, and they try to distance themselves from the patient. **Wariness and suspicion may become a part of the relationship.** Patients may begin to feel that there is no one that they can talk to about their illness.

4. Suicide

Fortunately for most patients, this is only a fleeting thought. Patients' lives have become so disrupted and disturbed that there can be little attraction in life. Each day, patients get up hoping to be cured. When this does not happen, they feel lost. Their friends and relatives do not appreciate the frustration. Rapidly, patients can become isolated and lonely. **The world may have little attraction. In this situation, contemplation** of suicide is not surprising and can even appear to be a logical solution to many problems. Fortunately, the vast majority of patients reject suicide. This is probably because PVFS patients usually have a great zest for life, and suicidal feelings can quickly pass.

5. Conclusion

Psychological problems, therefore can be an inherent part of PVFS. **However, psychological disorders are definitely not the cause of PVFS.** The symptoms and the length of illness may suggest to doctors that the patient has a psychiatric disorder, and indeed in some patients viral infections may precipitate anxiety and depression (British Journal of Psychiatry, 1976; 128 : 559-61). As the illness continues, the patient can develop more symptoms which can have the effect of making psychological problems worse. It is a vicious circle from which the patient needs to escape. **The first step involves patients maintaining their sanity by believing in themselves and adopting a plan for recovery.**

ASSOCIATED DISORDERS

1. Psychiatric Disorders

Psychiatric disorders are associated with PVFS. This means that in patients with PVFS a small number may develop a psychiatric disorder. Similarly, in patients with a psychiatric disorder a small number may develop PVFS. **Psychiatric disorders are not the cause of PVFS.** There are several other conditions which are associated with PVFS. The relationships between these syndromes and PVFS are depicted in Figure 12.

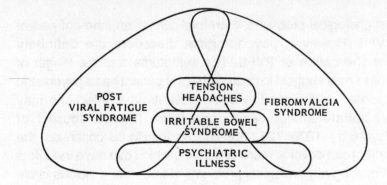

Figure 12   Conditions associated with PVFS
Patients with fibromyalgia syndrome, tension headaches, irritable bowel syndrome or psychiatric disorders may develop PVFS. This is probably because infection may occur in any group of patients. Similarly, patients with PVFS may go on to develop these associated conditions.

2. Fibromyalgia Syndrome

This is an illness in which there are very tender areas in characteristic sites in a patient's body. The illness is usually chronic and there is evidence that many patients have an abnormal sleeping pattern (Physician 1990 : 581-583). Medical practitioners can differentiate these two illnesses. **It is important to distinguish this condition from PVFS as the management is different.**

3. Tension Headaches

These are believed to be a result of stress on an individual. In individuals with tension headaches, fatigue is usually a minor complaint, and these patients can be completely well in the absence of stress. Patients with PVFS may develop such headaches and they may last weeks, and the headaches can be very resistant to treatment. **However, in PVFS the headaches are principally a result of over-activity, although stress may be an influential factor.** Headaches in PVFS are managed symptomatically and with bed rest.

4. Irritable Bowel Syndrome

The situation here is quite different. **A large number of PVFS patients have abdominal complaints especially alternating diarrhoea and contstipation.** In addition, abdominal "fullness" or "bloating" after a meal are common. In many patients the muscles in the gastrointestinal tract are probably affected. This problem is considered in greater detail in Chapter Twelve.

MANAGEMENT

Good days and bad days are a part of the illness. On good

days, patients can be high on top of a mountain. On bad days, descent into the sea of depression can apparently take hours (Figure 13). This need not happen, instead patients should plan for bad days. **We all have things that cheer us up and patients can take early actions to prevent falling into the sea of depression.**

These actions seem so trivial that they are often not even considered by the patient. **Yet, this approach works. The essence is to recognise that *early* action is required.** Patients should put aside a variety of obstacles to depression (Figure 13). These may be : favourite videos (especially cartoons); jokes that have been particularly funny; pets whose antics make you laugh; or, food that makes you happy, even if it is a special chocolate.

Recordings on a tape recorder or video of favourite programmes on radio or television are particularly useful. However, similar enjoyment may be obtained from looking at travel brochures, or reading a passage in a book about an odd place or situation. **Patients who are prone to becoming depressed should collect things that make them laugh.** An important aspect of managing patients with PVFS is to recognise the importance of laughter. **When people laugh their bodies function more effectively. There is evidence that the immune system is more effective, with greater circulation of natural killer cells.** These cells are the body's first line response to dealing with infection. Laughter can stimulate their production. **Some patients should laugh for five minutes, three times a day. It sounds a bit odd, but it works.**

For most patients prone to depression, these remedies can prevent deep depression. However for a number of patients, antidepressants are required (Chapter Thirteen). Patients

HIGH

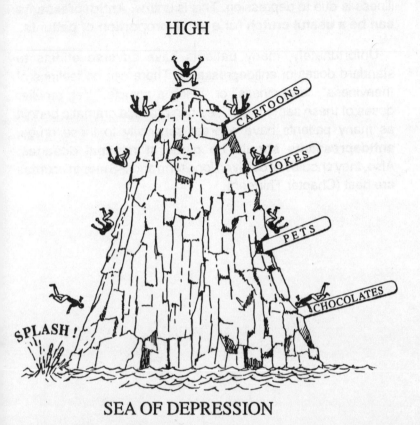

SEA OF DEPRESSION

Figure 13   Sea of depression
Many patients tumble down from a high at the top of a mountain into the sea
of depression. This need not happen. Instead, a choice of cartoons, jokes,
pets and even food (such as chocolate) can be effective obstacles to clinical
depression.

sometimes feel that they should not accept such therapy. They may feel that if they take antidepressants, it will prove that their illness is due to depression. This is untrue. **Antidepressants can be a useful crutch for a small proportion of patients.**

Unfortunately, many patients have adverse effects to standard doses of antidepressants. There can be feelings of "heaviness", "drowsiness" or "being a zombie." Yet, smaller doses of these same medicines can produce dramatic benefit as many patients have a great sensitivity to these drugs, **antidepressants should be given at minimal dosages.** Also, they should not be given long term and 3-6 month courses are best (Chapter Thirteen).

SUMMARY

1. Patients with PVFS have to believe in themselves. They must maintain their sanity, recognise that they are ill and adopt a plan for recovery.

2. The patients' emotional state may predispose them to viral infections and delayed recovery.

3. Fatigue (asthenia) or tiredness are common complaints of patients with psychiatric disorders. PVFS patients are easily distinguished from psychiatric patients by the case definition of PVFS.

4. Psychiatric disorders (depression, anxiety, paranoia, suicide) are often a result of the illness. PVFS is not caused by psychiatric disorders.

5. A number of conditions are associated with PVFS : psychiatric disorders, fibromyalgia syndrome, tension headaches and irritable bowel syndrome.

6. Patients should adopt strategies to prevent depression. They should collect things that make them laugh.

7. Antidepressants may be of great value to some patients. As patients are sensitive to these drugs, they should be given in low dosage.

CHAPTER EIGHT
SECOND STEP: ACQUIRE KNOWLEDGE

The tycoon who had taken over the company was ruthless. He could not accept criticism and always got his own way. He decided that he would introduce his own pension plan. On paper, his offer sounded great with benefits in all sections of the pension plan. His only stipulation was that all employees should accept it within 48 hours.

The employees were overjoyed and could not believe their good fortune. All signed quickly except Sid. His colleagues could not believe it and put tremendous pressure on Sid, but he simply said :
"It's too complicated and I don't understand it."

They tried everything but could not change his mind. With one hour to the deadline, the tycoon called Sid to his penthouse and said :
"Sid, the penthouse is on the twentieth floor of this building. If you do not sign the new pension plan before I count to ten, I will push you out the window."

Immediately, without waiting for the counting to start, Sid signed. The tycoon was not surprised but asked :
"Why did you not sign before"?
Sid paused, but then explained:
"You are the first person to explain why I had to sign".

Patients with PVFS need to acquire knowledge of their illness to recover. This is because their illness is individual and only the patient can truly understand the many individual facets of the illness. However, acquisition of knowledge is not easy (Table 8).

The five types of knowledge as stated in Table 8 will be further discussed in the rest of this chapter.

Table 8   Difficulty in acquiring knowledge

	Knowledge	Difficulty
1.	Illness (general)	Low
2.	Illness (detailed)	Medium
3.	Self	High
4.	Individual PVFS effects	High
5.	Answers to relapses	High

It is readily apparant that apart from general knowledge of the illness, none of these tasks are easy. Indeed, most tasks are of a high degree of difficulty. If a patient is able to acquire the knowledge, the next step is to apply the knowledge. **When knowledge is applied to the illness, patients can develop control of the illness.** With this control, there is a greater confidence and the realisation that recovery is possible. From this realisation, it is a short step to knowing that recovery will soon come.

GENERAL KNOWLEDGE

General knowledge of the illness is relatively easy to acquire. For many, this can be simply reading a newspaper or magazine article about the illness. Many patients are happy to just try to establish that the illness exists. **At this stage, they may feel that if they find any more information, they may be accused of wanting to be ill.** Sadly, the effects of the illness make people defensive.

Patients' perceptions of the illness can be illogical. Many times patients have admitted to me that they did not like the diagnosis of PVFS and would rather if I said that they had a cancer. **This atitude is totally different to the general public's belief that PVFS patients would choose the diagnosis of PVFS rather than be well.** This is yet another example of the divide between reality and its perception. Patients need to acquire professional status rather than continuing to be amateurs. They need to have detailed knowledge rather than what is generally available. **The problem is major; patients need to become serious.**

DETAILED KNOWLEDGE

Detailed knowledge of the illness is not easily acquired and involves a medium degree of difficulty. Patients will have to try and understand all of their symptoms. They will need to read a book about their illness. With this greater knowledge, patients will be able to see their illness as a whole. **Sadly many patients see their illness as only bad news** (Figure 14). It requires a great effort to even start to look for information with this attitude in mind.

Pope has said :

92

PATIENT'S LIFE

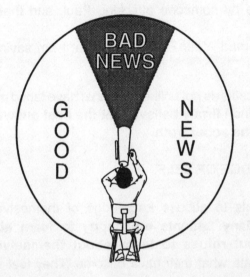

Figure 14 Patient's life

Many patients can only see the bad news in their illness. Patients can appear
to have limited vision. Part of recovery depends on patients being able to see
their illness as a whole. Many will then recognise that there is more good
news than bad news.

"A little learning is a dangerous thing; Drink deep, or taste not the Piorian spring". I once mentioned this quotation to a patient who replied by quoting from the bible :
"Too much learning doth make thee mad" (Acts 26:24).
It is perhaps instructive to remember that the above statement was made by someone attacking Paul, and that Paul had replied :
"I am not mad, Your Excellency, what I am saying is sober truth".

This situation is not unlike those that have faced many PVFS patients, and **I firmly believe that the best answers will be found in the sober truth.**

KNOWLEDGE OF SELF

For patients to acquire knowledge of themselves is very difficult. **Many patients are happy to learn about their illness, but refuse to learn about themselves.** Often, patients hate what they have become. They feel that if they acquire more knowledge of themselves, their worse fears will be confirmed. **Their worse fears are usually that they would not be able to be active again.**

Patients remember their past life and cannot bear to look at their present position. **They are essentially mourning the death of their past existence.** As with all mourning, their ability to face the facts is limited. They refuse to accept that their past existence is over. **Yet, for recovery, patients need to understand what is happening and recognise their mourning.**

Fortunately, for most patients their past existence is not as important as they perceive it. With time and honesty, it will be recognised that they often lived on adrenaline. As all drugs, it can be addictive. Yet, it is possible to be happy and content without adrenaline. **Recovery can depend on patients being able to recognise that in the past they depended on activity and adrenaline for a "high".**

INDIVIDUAL PVFS EFFECTS

When sufferers talk among themselves, they realise that they have great similarities as well as great differences in their illnesses. **It is very unusual to find two patients with exactly the same complaints.** This does not mean that different patients have different illnesses. Instead, it should be realised that a patient's complaints are individual (Figure 15). The illness has such widespread effects on the body that complaints are many and varied.

I am often amazed at the paradox of patients' perception of their past and current lives. In the past, they were productive, active and triumphed in their individuality. **Currently, as they are not productive or active, they want to be exactly the same as other sufferers.** The only way that they are the same as before is in their individuality, but they want to reject this only similarity with the past. It is a symptom of the lack of confidence that comes with illness. Somehow it is no longer possible to wear the scarlet tie or scarf.

ANSWERS TO RELAPSES

In most cases, relapses are not random. With a diary (Chapter Nine) it is possible to explain about 80% of relapses. Thus with knowledge it is possible to understand the illness. The great advantage of this understanding is that patients can feel that they are not being manipulated by random events. **They are not puppets on strings.** Instead, the effects are a

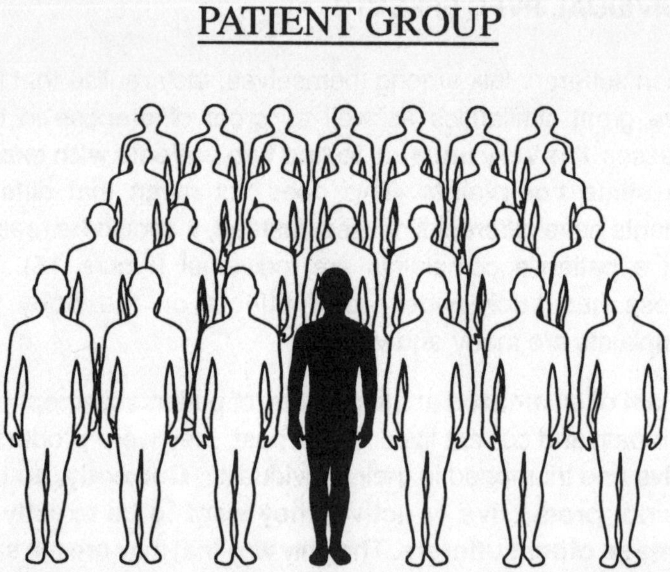

PATTERN GROUP

Figure 15   Patient group
In a large group of patients with PVFS, each patient's complaints will be slightly different. For each patient, the illness will have individual effects. This is why it is important for patients to acquire personal knowledge of their illness.

result of their behaviour or environmental factors (such as jobs, relatives, relationships and finances) around them (Chapter Eleven).

Understanding as a result of knowledge allows patients to predict how they will feel in the future. The ability to predict the future produces a feeling of control. **Slowly, patients start to develop their confidence again.** With greater confidence there is a feeling of well-being and progress. It is a great result but the process is slow.

SUMMARY

1. Patients often feel that if they acquire too much information about their illness, they may be accused of wanting to be ill.

2. Patients require to have detailed knowledge of their illness. Their illness is not only bad news and the best answers will be found in sober truth.

3. Patients often have fears of knowing themselves. Many mourn their past existence and believe that they have no worth when they are ill.

4. PVFS patients are individual and it is unusual to find two patients with the same complaints. Before illness, patients prided themselves on their individuality; with illness, patients want to be the same. It is a reflection of a loss of confidence.

CHAPTER NINE
THIRD STEP: A DAILY DIARY

Brian was a man who did not like to spend money. He was reknown for taking lemonade bottles back to the shop, and using candles instead of electric lights at night. Yet, Brian was a very handsome man, and beautiful women were immediately attracted to him. Unfortunately, after a short time, these women could not cope with his stinginess.

One day, he was waiting for a bus. When the bus finally arrived, he asked the conductor how much it was to the bus terminal.
"Fifty pence" said the conductor.
This was too much for Brian, so he decided to run behind the bus for the next two stops, and then asked :
"How much is it to the bus terminal now?" "Still fifty pence" replied the conductor.
Brian ran a further five stops - just to make sure that it would be cheaper and asked :
"How much is it now?"
"Eighty pence" said the conductor, "You're running in the wrong direction."

Many patients, even with the very best intentions, are running in the wrong direction. They are so close to their illness that it is impossible for them to see matters are getting worse. Most patients were previously well-organised individuals who prided themselves on their abilities to solve problems. Sadly, when memory and/or concentration are affected, a once efficient individual may behave like a headless chicken.

When people succeed in life, they often have an edge. It may be in ability, organisation or luck. Usually success is a reflection of accentuating one's strengths and minimising the effects of one's weaknesses. **It therefore makes sense to compensate for poor memory by keeping a daily diary.**

A daily diary is not easy to keep. Many patients and their relatives regard a daily diary as "patients wallowing in their illness." I cannot accept this argument. Recovery depends on knowledge; and without a diary, how do you know if you are running in the right direction? Patients often reply that they know that they are getting worse. **If patients are getting worse, they are obviously running in the wrong direction.**

There are several difficulties in keeping a daily diary (Table 9). These difficulties have to be approached in a systematic way, and it must be recognised that it will take time and effort to become a proficient diarist.

Table 9   Difficulties in keeping a daily diary

	Problem	Difficulty
1.	Desire	Great
2.	Format	Low
3.	Regularity	Medium
4.	Content	Low

99

5.	Precision	Medium
6.	Scoring system	Great
7.	Learning	Great

For an ill individual, Table 9 may appear formidable. Yet, overall it is not a difficult task - with help. **I have not found a patient who is unable to keep a good diary.** Indeed, many children can be taught to produce excellent diaries. However, patients must first want to help themselves.

1. DESIRE

Many patients initially accept the need for a diary, but after a week they cannot be bothered. **I feel that the diary is so important that I would refuse to see a patient who did not keep a diary.** Apart from the reasons given above, I can tell how a patient has been over six weeks in 5 minutes if the patient has a diary. If there is no diary, the same information takes 45-60 minutes to acquire. The desire to keep a diary is of high difficulty because patients have no energy to keep a diary, and they feel that their lives are so boring that there is no help in a diary. Patients often say "every day is exactly the same," "all I do is rest" or "I have no energy to do anything." Yet, some patients get better and others do not. **In patients who are getting worse, there is usually several things that they are doing wrong.** The fastest way for me to find out what they are doing wrong is to examine a daily diary.

   The daily diary that I like takes 3 minutes per day to keep. This is not a large amount of time. I believe that if patients cannot give 3 minutes per day for their diary, it is not surprising that they are not getting better. **The diary must also be written by the patient.** I am often told "my wife/husband will do the diary" or "my mother/father is good at writing." **However,**

I always insist on the patient doing the diary. Even young children can be taught to keep a useful diary. It is also a measure of the patient's commitment to getting better.

2. FORMAT

The format of the diary is depicted in Figures 16 and 17. **A school exercise book is best as you can write on both sides of the paper.** It is better than photocopying the format, although photocopying reduces some work, it is not as easy to refer to or use.

Two pages should be used for each week : one page for scores (Figure 16) and the next page for the patient's activities (Figure 17). The scoring system is explained later in this chapter. Sometimes patients feel that they want to write more. This is good but it is important that this diary be on one page, and often patients who like to write will keep two diaries. In another diary, they may go into greater detail and even record more private matters. **My agreement with patients is simply that they keep a daily diary.** It is of tremendous importantance and takes only 3 minutes per day.

3. REGULARITY

Initially, patients may write 2-3 pages in their diary when they are feeling well; and if they have a relapse there will be blank pages, they will reply with indignation :
"I did nothing, so I wrote nothing!" This is not good enough. **I only require two lines each day, but I need these two lines every day of the year.** If the daily diary is not kept, it is of limited use.

The format of my diary is designed to be simple. It can be done even though patients are very ill. Many patients remark

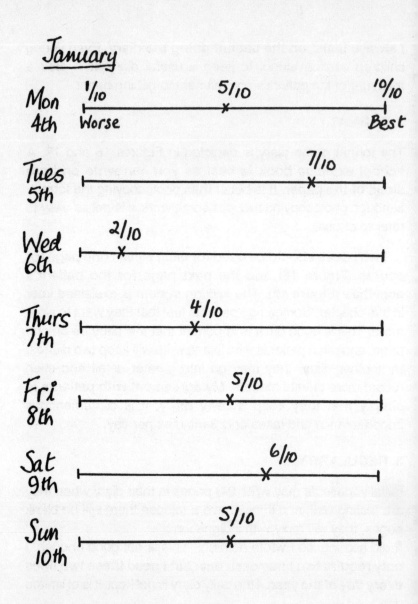

Figure 16 Left-hand page of the diary.
One page is used for each week. On the left-hand page of an exercise book,
daily scores are kept of how the patient feels on a scale of 1-10.

Mon Sleep 12 hrs. Hospital. Very tired
Sleep afternoon. TV. Bad day.

Tues Sleep 14 hrs. Good night. Long walk
Telephone x3. Visitors x2. Good day

Wed Sleep 8 hrs. Bad night. Very tired
No energy. Back to bed. Terrible.

Thurs Sleep 7 hrs. Disturbed. No energy.
TV. Relaxation(x2). Better day.

Fri. Sleep 12 hrs. Newspapers. Relaxation.
Telephone x1. Boring day.

Sat Sleep 14 hrs. Argument with mother.
Shopping 2 hrs. Telephone x2.

Sun Sleep 10 hrs. Church. Visitors x2
Relaxation x2. Unhappy day.

Figure 17 Right-hand page of the diary
One page is used for each week. On the right-hand page, two lines describe
the patient's day. Do not write in sentences. Record hours of sleep and
relaxation, activities, visitors, telephone calls, problems and how you feel.

at how simple the diary appears. Yet, this is usually when patients have a lot to say. The diary can be very difficult for an individual who is in relapse. **However, I have only rarely encountered a patient who is unable to keep a daily diary despite the seriousness of the relapse.** A daily diary is a cornerstone for better recovery.

4. CONTENT

Although this is of low difficulty (Table 9), many patients find this a problem. A major consideration is that many patients remember how active they were, in comparison and feel that there is nothing to write. Although such an approach is logical, it does not deal with the problem. **The problem is simply that without detailed daily information, a patient's chance of recovery is greatly diminished.**

It is easier if patients have a systematic approach to the content of a diary. Firstly, there is no need to write in sentences. It is only 2-3 lines and therefore it needs to contain as much information as possible. State the important facts first: hours of sleep, hours of relaxation and if you are having a period (menstruation). Next, record how you have spent your time if you have watched television, listened to the radio, read the newspapers or books, had visitors or made telephone calls. Lastly, say how you feel (happy, unhappy, good, bad etc). **Do not become discouraged about your diary.** With time, you will develop an understanding of what should be in the diary. Like many skills in life, a diary takes time and effort. The reward is better recovery from PVFS.

5. PRECISION

Many diaries start off being emotional rather than precise. Frequent comments are : "This is hell on earth," "I am about to die," "I've never experienced such torture," "When will I find peace?" and "The pain is unbearable." However, to be of value, a diary needs to be precise. So, more useful comments would be : "I can't get out of bed," "I can only walk 100 yards," "I had diarrhoea ten times today," or "My headache lasted 12 hours."

A precise diary allows comparison over time. One or two years later, patients may be able to go back and see how they were. I am always surprised that patients are quite happy to say to me :
"I have not been well for years and it is getting worse each year."
Yet, when I ask when it started, there is usually a blank stare. When I ask how has it got worse over each six-month period, there is a look of astonishment that I might require such information. **Without such information it is impossible to predict the future progress of the illness.**

6. SCORING SYSTEM

Patients need to have an overall impression of how they are. This takes time. The first difficulty is that patients feel differently at different times of the day. Some are worse in the morning; others are worse at night. Some patients often feel that they should score themselves in the morning, afternoon, evening and at night. This is too complicated. **Patients should learn to develop an overall average score for the day.** This is the easiest and most useful approach.

A rough guide to the scoring system is in Table 10. This table gives several guidelines. Although it appears very difficult, patients usually quickly learn to use a scoring system.

Table 10   The scoring system

Score	Effects
1.	Severe symptoms at rest. In bed all day.
2.	Moderate to severe symptoms at rest. Unable to work. Concentration and activity severely affected.
3.	Moderate symptoms at rest. Unable to work full-time. Activities severely affected.
4.	Mild symptoms at rest. May just be able to work full-time but not in a physical or stressful job. Frequent rest/relaxation needed.
5.	Very mild symptoms at rest. Moderate to severe symptoms with exercise or activity. Able to work full-time, but not in a physical or stressful job. Social life restricted.
6.	Very mild or no symptoms at rest. Moderate symptoms with exercise. Able to work full-time, but not in a physical job. Social life affected.
7.	Very mild or no symptoms at rest. Mild symptoms, with exercise. Able to work full-time but not in a physical job. Some social life.
8.	No symptoms at rest. Very mild or no symptoms with some exercise. Able to work full-time in a reasonably active job. Some social life.
9.	No symptoms at rest. Little symptoms with exercise. Able to work full-time in a reasonably active job. More social life.
10.	Patient well.

The scoring system is rated as being of high difficulty (Table 10). This is because there are several problems which patients have :

a) **Wanting to be precise :** using decimal places (5.1 or 4.25). Patients should stick to whole numbers, occasionally halves are acceptable.

b) **Changes in a week :** it is useful to look at a week and see one day that was better or worse than the rest. Thus, to see seven 5's is not as useful as five 5's, one 4 and one 6. Overall for the week the score is the same. Do not be afraid of using a range of numbers.

c) **Wanting to change past scores :** patients often say "last year this time I scored 5, but it was not really a 5, it was a 3; I am now a 5." The score that is correct is the score that you feel now. A year from now, if you feel better you should score yourself higher, rather than go back to the diary and change the previous year's scores.

d) **Fear of being too optimistic :** there is an irrational fear of scoring higher scores. It is not unlike the teacher who cannot give students full marks. The scoring system has guidelines (Table 10) but patients should score themselves relative to the previous days/weeks.

LEARNING

Patients usually do the diary because I ask them. **It is useful to me, but it should be more useful to the patient.** When the diary scores are bad, patients should do less. Thus the diary scores influence their behaviour in subsequent days. **Learning from the diary is the most difficult lesson.** Patients are often content to keep very detailed diaries, but not to let the diary influence their behaviour.

The diary is a key to answering many questions. Not all female patients feel worse during menstruation, but some do - the diary can provide the answer. One patient used the diary to realise that visiting her father made her worse. Another, detected a food allergy. **Patients need to use the diary to learn.**

CONCLUSION

Keeping such records can be demanding but they are necessary. A detailed diary shows an outsider that you are concerned about your illness and you are trying to be objective. But more important, a diary can be a tremendous boost when you are going through a difficult time. It is reassuring to be able to know how you compare to 1, 3 or 5 years ago. **Most patients over this period will have improved, although comparisons over shorter periods (weeks or months) may show deterioration.** The problems can also change with time and here a diary can be instructive. One patient was almost suicidal about her health and, from her diary, indicated that in a 3-year period she had had some ten different complaints. When it was pointed out that she had overcome 9 problems, her retort was a predictable "There were 9 too many!" **Being objective about one's illness is difficult. It takes time, and one does not know if it is worth it.** But what is the alternative? To sit around waiting for a miracle?

Detailed recording of symptoms is the third step to better recovery from viral infections. It reinforces and expands the first step which is deciding to become involved in one's illness. Specific knowledge about oneself will allow a change of attitude and lifestyle (details of which are in later chapters). **Great strength can come from the realisation that self-help is possible and that many solutions to problems are within one's capabilities.** Whereas recovery may take years, life can be better now. It just needs a positive start.

SUMMARY

1. A daily diary allows patients to know if they are making progress. It is the third step to better recovery.

2. It can be difficult to keep a daily diary, but first patients must want to record detailed information. The diary takes 3 minutes/day, and is not a long time for patients to devote to getting better.

3. Ideally, an exercise book should be used with two pages for each week. The diary should be kept daily. It should record the activities in the day, and a scoring system should be used.

4. The most important result of a daily diary is when a patient learns from the diary. The diary is not mainly for the doctor, but for the patient.

CHAPTER TEN
FOURTH STEP:
UNDERSTAND ENERGY I:
ACTIVITY AND SLEEP

In 1831, George Osbaldeston bet 1000 guineas that he could travel by horse faster than Stephenson's new Rocket locomotive. At the time, the Rocket travelled at the record speed of 24 miles per hour, and no one could see how Osbaldeston could win. Worse, the race was over 200 miles and Osbaldeston was handicapped. Forty-four years old, five foot tall with a badly crippled leg, he hardly looked capable of lasting the course. Amazingly, allowing for stops and riding 28 horses, he averaged 26 miles per hour and easily won his bet. At the end of the race, he announced that he was so hungry that he "could eat an old woman". Such feats of endurance have always had an attraction, and indeed, have a special section in the Guinness Book of Records.

Understanding energy is the most difficult step to better recovery. Patients think of energy as being active, and cannot usually think of ways of increasing their energy levels. **The**

major problem is that patients can only think of energy in terms of using it through activity. Because of this problem, over many years I have developed a strategy for teaching patients to understand energy (Table 11). The first three parts will be dealt with in this chapter and the last part in Chapter Eleven.

Table 11   Strategy for understanding energy

1. Think of energy as money
2. Energy lost by physical activity
3. Energy gained by sleep or relaxation
4. Energy lost by mental activity

ENERGY AS MONEY

The first part of the strategy is to think of energy as money. To get better, patients need to recognise that they cannot use more energy (or money) than they have. If they do, as with money, they will get worse (or go further into debt). Indeed, as patients are ill, they have a massive overdraft at the bank, so they need to save some money (or energy) each day. The first part of the strategy is explained in Figures 18 to 21. **My approach has worked with many patients over many years.** Yet, I am frequently asked why can you not exercise to recovery?

ENERGY LOST BY PHYSICAL ACTIVITY

Physical activity (exercise or work) is a very important part of life. It is not surprising that a frequent question is : how much exercise can I do?

Exercise itself is a complex subject, and as with religion, it means different things to different people.

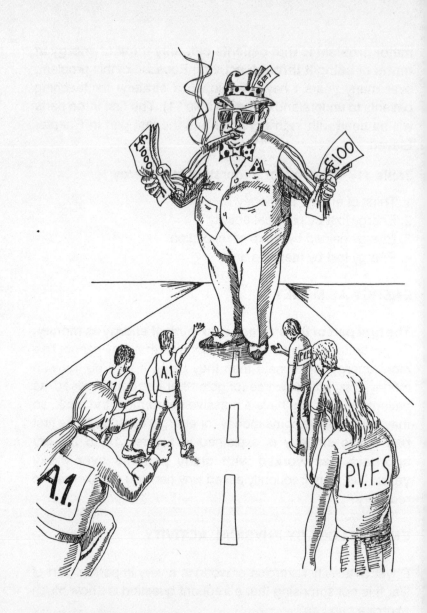

Figure 18   Energy as money

Patients should think that before the illness they had £1000 worth of energy for each day. With PVFS, they have £100 of energy for each day. Like someone losing their income, there has to be a severe cutback on activities.

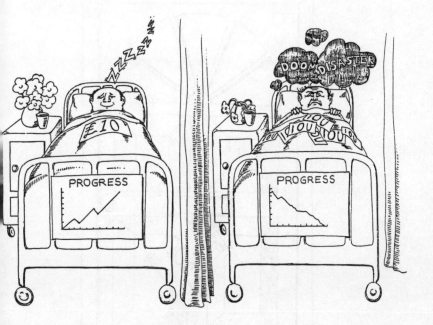

Figure 19 Progress on bad days

To make progress, patients have to go to bed with £10 unspent. For relapse
(doom and disaster), patients use more money (or energy) than they have
and end up borrowing money.

113

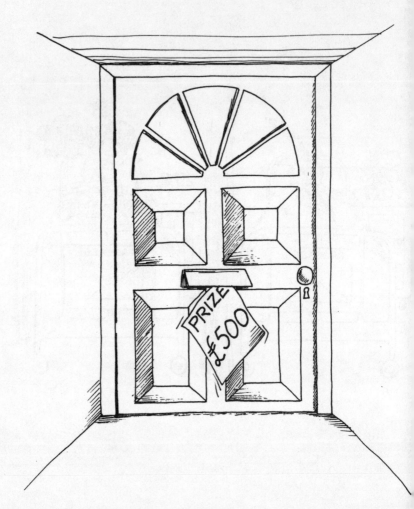

Figure 20   A Good Day
A good day is like having £500 worth of energy. It is like an unexpected prize
coming through the door.

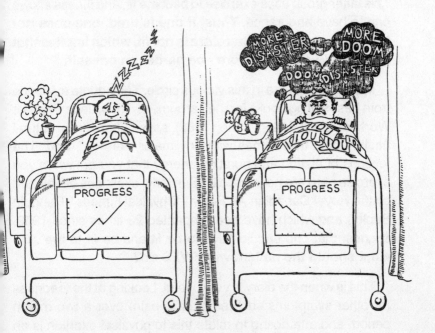

Figure 21   Progress on Good Days
To make progress on good days, patients should spend £300 and say that the amount is three times the bad days, and save £200. This repays the debt quicker and leaves something for tomorrow. Instead, patients usually try to catch-up with activities, spend all of the £500 and end up borrowing more money. Greater doom and disaster is inevitable.

Some equate exercise with activity which may be minimally energetic, such as taking the dog for a stroll to the shops. To others, exercise means endurance and "going for the burn". This latter group uses exercise to become fit, and fitness allows one to have endurance. **Thus, if one is tired, one does not have endurance, and therefore is not fit, which implies that one should exercise more - be harder on oneself.**

Many patients are in this vicious circle. They quote evidence from best-selling books for their argument. Thus, Jane Fonda's Workout Book (Allen Lane, 1982) says "There is a natural healthy pain that comes with any major exertion", and "The feelings of elation and bursting energy that you get when you exercise hard are not mystical". Similarly, exercises developed by the Royal Canadian Air Force ("Physical Fitness", Penguin Books) and which have been reprinted 23 times since 1958, suggest that one should "Live to be fit and be fit to live". **So what should the patient with PVFS do?**

This is when the diary is very useful. Looking at the tiredness (or other symptoms such as muscle pain) over a two month period, and attempting to relate this to physical exertion is an instructive lesson. In most patients, it is found that mild exercise, such as a 10 minutes walk or a 5 minutes swim, does not result in symptoms. Whereas, a hill walk for more than an hour, excessive physical activity, or lifting heavy weights can result in 2-7 days of tiredness. **With greater exercise other symptoms can also occur,** especially pain or burning in the muscles, diarrhoea, headaches, difficulty in seeing or hearing, and muscle twitches or tremors.

With the help of the diary, one can establish how much exercise can be tolerated and for how long. **The most important fact to realise is that - there is a considerable difference in what patients used to be able to do and what**

they can do now. For example, one patient enjoyed running 5 miles to work before his illness, but was only able to walk 100 yards without symptoms after his illness started. Many patients ignore their symptoms, and try to do exactly what they were capable of before their illness. The result is predictable, they feel unwell for the next 7-10 days. **Such forlorn attempts to emulate past achievements always take their toll.**

The difficulty patients have is recognising that they are ill. If one's leg was in plaster, no one would contemplate running 5 miles, but because there are no obvious physical signs of illness patients forget that they are ill. Like those around them, they have fallen into the trap of equating physical disability with illness. **The truth is that health is a reflection of what the body is capable of doing.** Wellbeing is not what the body looks as though it can do, or what someone thinks that it should do.

It is appropriate, here, to consider two other quotations. From "Physical Fitness" : "Although you may get some benefit from doing exercises until 'it hurts', this is not necessary in order to acquire an adequate level of physical fitness". And, if the quotation from Jane Fonda's book is completed : "There is a natural healthy pain that comes with any major exertion. The burn I talk about is that kind of pain. **There is also the pain that tells you something is wrong. Learn to listen to your body. It will tell you when there is a problem. And learn to read your pain".**

Generally patients do not benefit from increasing exercise until they are 80% recovered. It is as though the body needs to recover in other ways before exercise can produce a benefit. **The second part of the strategy (Table 11) is to learn that energy is lost by physical activity.**

TYPE OF ACTIVITY

Apart from the quantity and duration of physical activity, there is the type of activity. **Some activities use more money (energy) than others, so that the hour of squash is more exhausting than an hour of walking the dog.** Similarly, particular muscle groups can become overworked, so that half an hour chopping down a tree can have a more prolonged effect than the same time in the swimming pool. Team games in particular may require bursts of physical activity. **In general the best type of exercise is one in which the exertion is constant, and capable of being controlled by the patient.** Thus team games are not advisable, as it is usually not possible to go more slowly or stop. The best activity is one in which the patient controls the pace, however slow it may be.

Certain types of exercise, especially social ones tend to occur at the weekends. This can produce more noticeable effects. A patient with two exercise periods a week complained of excessive tiredness on Monday of each week. On further questioning, all of his activity was on Saturday and Sunday. When he changed his pattern to Saturday and Wednesday, his tiredness was dramatically reduced.

Muscle groups that were previously well-developed (e.g. arms or legs; right-handedness or left-handedness) tend to be more severely affected. **Similarly, activities that an individual used to be good at are often more tiring than entirely new activities.** Human behaviour is such that when times are bad, there is a tendency to dig-in or fall-back (i.e. repeat current activity or go back to activities in the past). Both of these natural instincts may result in more tiredness than developing a new interest.

It can be helpful to look upon the body as a rechargeable

battery. In the early stages of illness, it is a battery that cannot hold its charge for very long. Thus, exercise quickly results in exhaustion, and is followed by a prolonged period during which the body recharges itself. As the illness progresses, the body gradually improves and becomes a battery capable of holding its charge longer. Now, more exercise can be endured. **Exercise does not result in immediate tiredness, but often several days later, and recovery from tiredness is much faster.**

Ideally, the patient develops a feel for how much activity and the type of activity that can be tolerated. With the simile of the battery, he knows how much charge is going to be used with each activity, and what the effects will be. There are times when he decides to exhaust himself in the knowledge that recovery may take weeks. **These decisions are no worse than someone deciding to finish the punch at a party, and knowing that there will be a giant hangover the next day.**

EXERCISE TO RECOVERY?

Exhortations to fitness are only applicable to those with normal muscle function. All physical fitness books state this. "If you are in doubt as to your capability to undertake this programme see your medical practitioner." ("Physical Fitness") or Jane Fonda's book "You also have to consider any physical problems you have". **In the light of scientific evidence of abnormal muscle function, the advice must be against excessive exercise.**

As most individuals who develop PVFS appear to be more athletic than normal, it is not surprising that they should look upon exercise as a solution to their problems. **In the past, they remember being fit - a time when they were able to**

exercise vigorously, and feel the better for it. Worse, activities of the past are more likely to produce discomfort than a new activity. The crucial consideration is : in the past, their muscles behaved normally; but now, with PVFS their muscles are abnormal. **For the first six months, the advice must be: no strenuous exercise and remain within your energy limits no matter how difficult this may be.**

After the first six months, minor activity may help. This is good for morale. Short swims or walks are best. **The emphasis is on starting very, very slowly.** The muscles may take years to return to normal, so that the patient may never get past the stage of minor exertion. Advice from fitness books is consistent with this view. From "Physical Fitness" : "Start any training programme at a low level of activity and work up by easy stages". And Jane Fonda : "Give your body a chance to rev up again" after a break, also "When you develop your own exercise programme, listen to your body." Unfortunately for patients with PVFS, they may take years to progress further than the warm-up exercises. **If care is taken to record the recurrence, or worsening of symptoms in relation to exercise then patients will be able to determine for themselves the correct level of activity.**

SYMPTOMS

The usual symptoms are easy fatigue and excessive tiredness after minimal exertion. Exercise results in burning, hotness, or pain in various muscles especially the limbs. In some patients, other muscles are principally affected. Thus pain or tightness of the chest muscles or abdominal discomfort is common. Muscle dysfunction can express itself as tremors, twitches and uncoordinated movements; and more general symptoms such as dizziness, lightheadedness, headaches and diarrhoea can all occur after severe exercise.

The diary is particularly useful in showing relationships between symptoms and preceding events. It is best not to think of exercise as producing particular symptoms. **Whatever complaint the patient usually has is made worse by excessive exercise.** Exercise is an additional stress to the body and results in symptoms related to the activity, and worsening of existing complaints. Using the analogy of the battery, if the inside car lights are dim because of a poorly-charged battery, these lights become dimmer when the headlights are on full-beam.

It is important to record precise symptoms and to note if they recur with all types of activity. One patient, an avid DIY enthusiast, reported headaches and feeling faint after one hour of painting the house. These complaints only occurred with painting and not with walking or gardening. On further examination, it was found that the patient was reacting to the paint fumes. Thus, it was not the physical exertion of painting that caused his symptoms, but rather his sensitivity to the paint fumes (which may have been due to his PVFS). Because the symptoms in PVFS are so extensive, it is mandatory that other causes be looked for. The reason for this is that these other causes are often a lot easier to treat.

CAUSE OF TIREDNESS

What is the cause of excessive tiredness in PVFS? Two popular answers have been suggested. The first is that the body is weak so tires easily (because of exhaustion), as the patient is unfit. The second is that the body takes a long time to return to normal (because of delayed recovery), again due to the patient being unfit. Thus, many patients conclude that their tiredness is due to them being unfit; and if they became fit again, their tiredness would go away. In patients with PVFS, there is no evidence to support this conclusion. **This reasoning is only applicable in those with normal body function. The evidence in patients with PVFS is that their body function is abnormal - they are ill.**

In normal muscles, pain (or the burn) is due to the build up of lactic acid. Jane Fonda says of this : "There is absolutely nothing harmful or dangerous about it. It just slows you down until the oxygen supply is replenished, which is a matter of seconds." Using the technique of magnetic resonance imaging (Lancet 1984; i: 1367-9) in PVFS, the muscles have been shown to form lactic acid more quickly and to take longer to get rid of it as compared to normal. The excessive accumulation of lactic acid is probably a result of disordered metablolic regulation in the muscles - a result of the viral infection. **Thus, in patients with PVFS, the reason for this tiredness is both exhaustion and delayed recovery.** Neither are caused by the patient being unfit, but rather, by the muscles behaving abnormally.

There is additional evidence of muscle abnormality. Single fibre electromyography has shown atypical results in PVFS (Journal of Neurology, Neurosurgery and Psychiatry, 1985; 48: 691-94). Another paper has suggested that patients may have a partial deficiency in oxidative phosphorylation (Australian and New Zealand Journal of Medicine, 1985; 15 : 305-8). These early reports are promising, but cannot yet be used diagnostically. Also, not all patients demonstrate the same abnormalities, as there are likely to be several mechanisms which result in muscle dysfunction.

SLEEP

Sleep gains energy and is the fourth part of the strategy for understanding energy (Table 11). The public perceives good sleep to be : instant sleep as the head touches the pillow; total unconsciousness for eight hours; and no vivid dreams. In particular, it is considered to be very poor sleep if one wakes often during the night. It is not recognised that this concept of sleep has been learnt : babies do not sleep through the night, and in terms of survival it makes more sense to wake frequently.

In the past, people were also able to vary their sleeping hours with the seasons of the year. Thus in winter, they would sleep 14-16 hours and thus have less need for food, warmth or light. Whilst in the summer, they would sleep 4-6 hours and make use of the daylight.

Everyone dreams every night. Again, we have been taught to forget our dreams. When faced with a child having had a vivid dream, parents often say, "Never mind, go to sleep and forget the dream." Similarly, "It was only a dream, think of something else". The teaching to the child is that dreams are not important and should be forgotten. With PVFS, sleep is disturbed, variable (4-16 hours) and vivid dreams are common. These are all normal findings and should not be a source of worry. **I am happy if patients are in bed for 10 hours with their eyes closed, and not listening to the radio or music.** I do not worry about how often they wake or their vivid dreams.

A constant complaint of patients is the increased amount of sleep that they require. For some, double the sleeping time still does not seem to be enough. Others try to stop themselves sleeping as they fear "sleeping their lives away". It is important to realise that there is a reason for sleep. **Sleep, unlike fat, is**

not stored in the body. The analogy with fat is instructive. Many patients only experience of being responsible for their own health is in the control of their weight. To remove fat one stops eating. Thus, it seems logical if one sleeps too much, to stop sleeping. **But, one sleeps to recover from the past and not to prepare for the future.**

Restrictions on sleep make matters worse. **A catastrophic double is if a patient decides to "snap" out of his condition by excessive exercise and reduced sleep.** This is like getting a £10,000 loan to repay a debt, burning the money and wondering why there is no improvement in the financial position. **During sleep, there is healing of damaged body tissues** (British Medical Journal, 1984; 289: 1400-1) and there is reduced breakdown of muscle cells. Thus, through sleep the body is not only able to increase the rate of repair of damaged tissues, but also to reduce the rate of breakdown of normal tissues. **It is an attempt by the body to make itself better. Avoidance of sleep delays the repair of muscles.** One should not be afraid to sleep.

Patients should also understand sleep cycles. Thus, there are natural cycles at 20-30 mins and at 90 mins. If patients awake at these times, they feel refreshed. However, if patients awake at 60 mins, they feel more tired and convinced that sleep makes them worse. **Sleep can be curative.** It may be helpful to remember Shakespeare's words of Macbeth :

"Sleep that knits up the ravell'd sleave of care,
The death of each day's life, sore labour's bath,
Balm of hurt minds, great nature's second course,
Chief nourisher in life's feast."

RELAXATION

Relaxation is often used to mean "not being active", "sitting in front of the television", "resting", or "recreation". **For PVFS patients, relaxation can be an active process which creates more energy.** To achieve this end, a relaxation technique needs to be learnt. Such a technique, **EMBME** (entrance, muscles, breathing, mind and exit), has been extensively described ("Unwind" by Dr Darrel Ho-Yen, Dodona Books, 1991).

The last part in the strategy of understanding energy is the recognition that energy is lost by mental activity (Table 11). This is such an important concept it is dealt with separately in the next chapter (Chapter Eleven).

MAKING ENERGY LAST

It is difficult to make energy (and money) last. When people lose their job, it can be a long time before they adjust to their reduced circumstances. Instead, they continue to spend as before, hoping to be employed soon. **The position is similar to PVFS patients, and as with unemployment, those individuals who adjust best, do so early.** Patients need to live within their budget (energy and money) now.

If one gave a group of people £10 to spend on food for a week, there will be a variety of responses. Some would not be able to feed themselves for one day; others would be able to eat for two weeks. Similarly, PVFS patients have to learn the skill of making money (energy) last.

This is greatly helped if patients slow the day down and develop a routine. Working people have breakfast, read the papers and listen to the radio or television at the same time, all in 30 minutes. **This uses up a lot of energy as it requires a lot of concentration. For patients, these should be separate activities.** Thus, patients should have breakfast (30 minutes), make coffee and drink it slowly (30 minutes), read the papers (30 minutes) and then listen to the radio or television (30 minutes). **What previously took 30 minutes should now take 2 hours; it uses less energy and makes available resources last.**

Patients will also need to spend their time in different ways. **Television and videos are not recommended as they can use much energy.** It is better for patients to develop interests which do not take much concentration. **Thus, listening to music, especially classical, operatic or native, can be very uplifting.** Similarly, pets (such as fish or a bird) can be observed for hours on end.

SUMMARY

1. Patients need to develop a strategy for understanding energy.

2. They should think of : energy as money; energy is lost by physical activity; energy is gained by sleep and relaxation; and energy is lost by mental activity.

3. Patients with PVFS need to use only the energy (money) that they have.

4. Different types of activity use more/less energy. Activities may result in symptoms days later.

5. The cause of tiredness is not unfitness, but that PVFS has resulted in the body not behaving in a normal manner. The patient is ill.

6. All complaints can be made worse by excessive activities. New complaints may also develop.

7. Sleep can be curative, and should not be resisted. It allows the body to heal itself. There are many misconceptions about sleep.

8. Relaxation is an active process which creates more energy.

9. Patients need to learn to make energy last.

CHAPTER ELEVEN
FOURTH STEP: UNDERSTAND ENERGY II: STRESS AND RELATIONSHIPS

It was the best restaurant in the country. The dining-room was small and intimate. The atmosphere was perfect : the tables were not too close together and the lighting allowed you to see the food. But even better, the food was good and the restaurant had consistently won all the top awards for the last 10 years. Inevitably, it was expensive, No, it was very, very expensive. Nevertheless, it seemed just the place to see Ann Woods, a businesswoman who had built up her company over 20 years so that it now employed 500 people.

The chauffeur had parked the Mercedes and Ann was sitting at the best table in the restaurant. She had just ordered the most expensive meal on the menu and each course was accompanied by the finest wines. Just then, a friend who was leaving saw Ann and was obviously surprised at seeing her alone.
"It's my 25th wedding anniversary" replied Ann.

Her friend was in a hurry and did not want to pursue matters, but added :

"How are you?"

"I am fine" replied Ann "But business is bad. I am nearly bankrupt"

Her friend was a bit taken aback and said :

"Oh come on Ann! It can't be all bad. You are in the best restaurant in the country. You have just ordered the most expensive meal with the finest wines. On top of it all, your marriage has lasted 25 years despite all the difficulties of your running your own business. Most women would be content with what you have got."

Ann shook her head and ruefully replied :

"Yes, but last year I could afford to bring my husband."

Relationships are one of the most important things in life, and are also very easy to get out of perspective. **It is easy for good relationships to be taken for granted, or for one to spend too much time in bad relationships.** Inevitably, relationships are about emotion and energy. PVFS patients can have great difficulty coping with relationships, simply because they take up so much energy.

The fourth step to better recovery is to understand energy. This is in two parts: activity and sleep (Chapter Ten); and, stress and relationships. **Relationships are emotional and therefore use up a lot of energy, thereby putting patients under a lot of stress.** Often, patients before their illness would have coped well with these relationships, but find great difficulties with illness. It is simply that too much energy is required.

STRESS

There is a particular definition of stress that I like : **stress is a process in which the resources of the person are matched against the demands of the environment.** In my book, "Unwind" (Dodona Books, 1991), stress management techniques are carefully considered. Simply, for chronically ill patients, to cope with stress requires either reducing the demands of the environment or increasing their resources. **Resources can be increased by sleep and relaxation techniques.** Unfortunately, time spent on relaxation techniques can be perceived by the patient to be boring (Figure 22).

Reducing the demands of the environment is much more difficult. Usually such demands are in three main areas: relationships, job and finances. Employment and finances are considered in Chapter Fourteen. Relationships will be considered as in Table 12. The energy needs in Table 12 are approximate. Obviously, a particularly annoying friend or relative can use up more energy than a partner. The table is a reflection of how I believe you should use your energy. **Thus, your partner should have most of your energy, followed by your family and lastly your friends.** Often, there is not enough energy for all, and patients have to choose their priorities.

Table 12   Stress and relationships

	Relationships	Stress	Energy Needs
1.	Friends	Low/medium	Low/Medium
2.	Relatives	Medium	Medium
3.	Family	High	High
4.	Partners	Very High	Very High

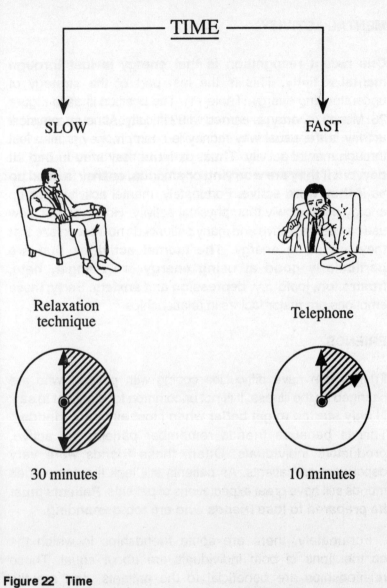

Figure 22   Time

When patients are performing a relaxation technique, time goes slowly and
30 minutes may appear to be 1 hour. However, when they are on the
telephone, time goes fast and 1 hour may appear to be 10 minutes. Patients
should spend no more than 10 minutes on one telephone call.

MENTAL ACTIVITY

One recent recognition is that energy is lost through mental activity. This is the last part of the strategy of understanding energy (Table 11). The position is as in Figure 23. Money (energy) is earned with difficulty. Although physical activity is the usual way money is spent, money is also lost through mental activity. **Thus, patients may stay in bed all day, but if they are worrying or anxious, energy is used up as if they were active.** Fortunately, mental activity uses up energy more slowly than physical activity. However, the slow use can be deceptive and many patients do not recognisze that they are using energy. **The mental activities that are particularly good at using energy are : anger, hate, frustration, jealousy, depression and anxiety.** Sadly, these emotions are major factors in relationships.

FRIENDS

Friends can have difficulties coping with patients who are changed by the illness. It is not uncommon for a patient to say: **"I only started to get better when I lost all of my friends."** This is because friends remember patients as active, productive individuals. Often, these friends were very dependent on patients. As patients still look the same, their friends still have great expectations of patients. **Patients must be prepared to lose friends who are too demanding.**

Fortunately, there are some friendships in which the contributions of both individuals are about equal. These relationships are beneficial to the patients, and are the friendships that should be continued. There is a simple test. **One feels better after sharing some time with a good friend.** If you are angry, annoyed or frustrated after being with

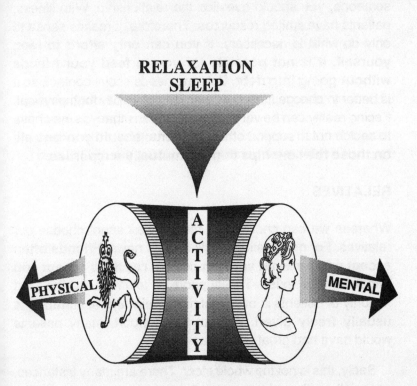

Figure 23   The ten pence coin
Sleep and relaxation earn money. The two sides of the ten pence coin show
how money is spent. The lion represents physical activity, and equally the
head represents mental activity.

someone, you should question the relationship. With illness, patients have limited resources. Therefore, it makes sense to only do what is necessary. **If you can only afford to feed yourself, it is not possible for you to feed your friends without going into debt.** But, one needs social contact, so it is better to choose friends who are happy to pay for their meal. Facing reality can be very difficult. It means that you may have to decide not to support others. **Patients should concentrate on those relationships that are mutually supportive.**

RELATIVES

Whereas we can choose our friends we cannot choose our relatives. For most patients, this is good news. **Friends often accept you for what you can do, but relatives accept you because you exist.** The support of relatives for the vast majority of patients is overwhelming. **Help and assistance is usually freely given.** Without this support, many patients would have had great difficulties.

Sadly, this is not the whole story. There are many instances, especially with a daughter and an older parent, where the relationship is unhealthy. **Several ill patients feel compelled to support an older parent.** In many cases, patients feel that it is their duty. There are usually tremendous feelings of guilt. Often, the parent manipulates the patient and makes many unreasonable demands. The patient dreads visiting the parent and would feel terrible after each visit. **My advice to these patients is simple : explain the situation to the parent and reduce the contact; do not feel guilty and do not be manipulated.**

Parents have a responsibility to care for their children; children do not have a responsibility to care for their

parents. If children care for their parents, they should do so for love and not because of guilt. Many patients have said to me that they hated their parents; yet, they were prepared to care for the parent, thereby prolonging their illness. I have sadly concluded that if a parent has manipulated offspring for more than 30 years, it cannot stop when the offspring become ill. **Worse, when the offspring is ill, he/she is least able to withstand the demands of parents.**

THE FAMILY

Under this section, I am considering the immediate family. **For patients, the family unit can determine whether they recover or not.** The support of the family is invaluable, and fortunately the goodwill in the family is usually high. This goodwill is the key to being able to use the resources of the family.

With illness, the patient's role within the family has to change. No longer is it possible for the mother to do all of the housework, or the father to do the handyman jobs about the house. The whole family have to be recruited to help. Children, even as young as five years, can be taught to be helpful. The great obstacle is accepting that the job will not be done properly. However, it is better for the children to clean the kitchen 60% as well as the patient. **The patient needs to accept this help, and gently teach the children.** I have felt that with time and good teaching, the job can even be done better than with the patient. With all good teaching the pupil should perform better than the teacher.

For those patients with a PVFS child their role needs considerable modification. Despite the difficulties, they will have to ensure that the child undertakes the programme as described in this book. Even the keeping of the diary must be entrusted to the child. I have found that children of 5-7 years can learn to keep a diary. There will be a need to modify some of the advice, but essentially children are managed in a similar way as adults. **The child must learn about the illness and take responsibility for his/her behaviour.** It is very difficult, but possible. As has been recognised over the centuries, in certain situations children can act in a remarkably responsible fashion. **In my experience, most problems arise when parents try to protect the child.**

PARTNERS

Partners (or **carers**) have a heavy, heavy burden. They see loved ones going through dramatic change : the active become inactive; the confident become afraid; the dependable become erratic; tears, anger and frustration become an everyday occurrence. For many it can be too much. **Many patients with PVFS end up separated or divorced.** However, I am impressed at how many relationships survive and prosper.

The relationships that do well have several common characteristics (Table 13). These characteristics are probably necessary for all good relationships, however, with illness they can become vitally important.

Table 13   Difficulties for a partner

	Characteristic	Difficulty
1.	Mutual respect	Low
2.	Consideration	Low
3.	Understanding	Medium
4.	Common objectives	Medium
5.	Time together	High
6.	Sexual activity	Very high

In Table 13, I have not mentioned love, possibly because it is so hard to define. **If love is present many of the characteristics are also present, and the relationship will be good.** However, in many relationships in which there is said to be love, one finds one partner doing all of the loving and the other consenting to be loved.

A good test of a relationship is the sexual activity, and in patients with PVFS this has a very high degree of difficulty. **There are substantial differences between men and women.** With men, sexual activity is generally regarded as the main course of a three course meal; without the main course, there is no sustenance. With women, sexual activity is generally regarded as the dessert of a three course meal; sustenance is obtained with the main course, and the dessert is consumed if there is still hunger, time and inclination. **Couples need to rethink their sexual activity depending on which partner is affected.** This is a matter of great importance and cannot be left until a patient recovers.

A good sexual relationship is an aid to recovery, and a poor one is a large hinderance. Success depends on sexual activity when there is energy and the time is right. This usually means that sex is better in the morning or after lunch rather than at night. It should not be rushed, patients need time for arousal.

It is a mistake to think of only touching each other during sexual activity. Often, there are good reasons for this, such as a patient being in a lot of pain. However, if there is love a gentle touch can be a powerful analgesic, cuddles should also be part of a healthy relationship, and need not necessarily lead to the sexual act. Many women find greater enjoyment out of cuddles compared to the sexual act.

Muscle and joint pain can be obstacles to sexual activity. Gentle massage of the affected partner is often a great prelude to sex and can reduce pain. Couples will also need to experiment with various sexual positions. Side by side can be a useful position, and do not be afraid of using pillows to support tender areas such as the neck or lower back. **Couples should experiment and be open in their discussion of each experiment.**

If the patient is the man, the situation is slightly easier. Some patients find it difficult to maintain an erection, but matters are helped if the woman is first well-lubricated. Again, a useful position is with the woman on top. **Both partners will need to develop great patience.**

When the patient is a woman, there may be a need to consider sex differently. Most women consider quality rather than quantity. Whereas, men would usually prefer to eat bread regularly rather than starve apart from feasts on good days. A solution is for the patient to masturbate the man between feasts. **In these circumstances, it is an act of giving and sharing.** It can keep a relationship alive and can be enjoyable to both partners.

Sadly, in some situations sexual intercourse is not possible. Some men may develop severe prostatitis and ejaculation can be very painful. Similarly, some women can find the sex act too painful. In these situations, masturbation of the partner should be considered. Fortunately, these circumstances are uncommon. **Indeed, some patients find orgasm as the one activity that totally relieves their symptoms.** This is probably because of the release of adrenaline and endorphins, but unfortunately the effects are short-lived and much energy is consumed in the process. Yet, sex is important for all relationships and should have a high priority because of its great benefits.

SUMMARY

1. Good relationships should not be taken for granted, and patients should not spend time and energy in bad relationships.

2. Relationships are emotional and use up energy through mental activity. They also create much stress. The amount of stress and energy varies with the type of relationship.

3. A ten pence coin should remind patients that energy is lost through physical and mental activities.

4. Patients may need to lose all of their friends before they can get better.

5. Relatives can be supportive. Some older parents may be unduly demanding on patients. Patients should not feel guilty about their parents.

6. The family unit can determine whether a patient recovers. The patient's role within the family will have to change and help will have to be accepted.

7. For patients with PVFS children, the parental task is difficult. Yet the child will have to be taught responsibility for his/her behaviour. It can be done with effort and patience.

8. Partners have an almost impossible task. For relationships to survive, several characteristics are necessary with sexual activity being the most difficult.

9. Couples need to rethink their attitudes and to experiment in their sexual activities.

CHAPTER TWELVE
FIFTH STEP : FOOD AND DIETS

"Let food be your medicine and medicine your food". This advice is attributed to Hippocrates, a Greek physician who practised medicine some 400 years before the birth of Christ. For his many writings and accurate observations, he has been called the "Father of Medicine". But perhaps the best indication of the high regard his fellow doctors had for him, was the adoption of his medical ethics in the "Hippocratic Oath" which is taken by every doctor on graduation.

The health properties of food have been recognised for thousands of years. The slaves who were assigned to building the giant pyramids were given daily doses of garlic to prevent illness. Subsequently, the Roman Empire is said to have survived without doctors with the help of the common cabbage. This lowly vegetable has great nutritional properties apart from being a useful wound dressing.

For PVFS patients, some understanding of food and diets is the fifth step to better recovery. The vast majority of patients need only consider the food section of this chapter.

For those with particularly worrying abdominal complaints, especially those who have been ill for many years, the section on diets may help.

FOOD

Health is made up of the triad of activity, food and sleep (Figure 24). **Matters are changed with illness when food is required for healing rather than activity.** It is important for all ill patients to have sufficient protein (meat, fish), carbohydrates (bread, rice), vitamins and minerals (vegetables and fruits). Fortunately, most patients living as part of a family are likely to eat well. **Smaller more frequent meals and eating the major meal in the middle of the day can also be particularly helpful.**

Patients who have been ill under one year should not worry too much about diets. They should simply attempt to eat normally. Problems are likely to occur when patients live alone because there is the temptation to miss meals. Patients often say that they are not hungry and have no energy to cook. **If a patient is *not* eating normally then major problems may arise.**

Vitamins are present in fresh fruit and vegetables. Vitamin tablets may be purchased and can be expensive. Patients often feel the need to take extra vitamins, not unlike buying a "tonic". **On the whole, most patients do not require extra vitamins.** Patients who are living alone and not eating normally may benefit from extra vitamins.

DIETS

Concern about food and dieting is now a national pastime. From the Pineapple Beverley Hills Diet to the F-Plan Diet,

HEALTH

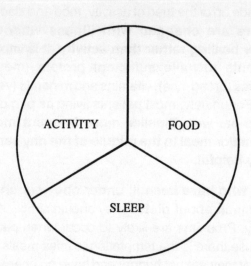

Figure 24   Health
For a healthy life, there are three main requirements : activity to occupy your
time; food for your daily activities; and sufficient sleep for your body.

142

Cambridge Diet and the High Carbohydrate and Fibre Diet ("Lean means beans"), the prime concern seems to be to lose weight in an unusual manner. Usually, the basis for the diet is not good scientific research, but rather the current fashion. Even the diets with an authentic past (macrobiotics, biogenics) are open to public opinion and fashion.

Most individuals diet to lose weight. This is not the position for some PVFS patients. **For patients with severe abdominal complaints or illness for many years, they diet to feel better.** Sadly, there are many available diets, and some of these diets require large amounts of time (Figure 25). **If you cannot find the time and energy to eat normally, you do not have sufficient time or energy for a diet.** The **anti-candida** diet has many advocates. It is very time consuming and can be quite expensive. I do *not* feel that most patients benefit from this diet. **I would rather patients take the time and effort to understand energy** (Chapter Ten and Eleven). In my experience this understanding is far more likely to produce recovery.

The diet that I have found most helpful to patients is the **"Hay System"**. This is superbly explained in "Food Combining for Health" by Doris Grant and Jean Joice (1984, Thorsons). There are five major rules :

a) starches and sugars should not be eaten with proteins and acid fruits at the same meal
b) vegetables, salads and fruits should form the major part of the diet
c) proteins, starches and fats should be eaten in small quantities
d) refined, processed foods should be avoided
e) an interval of 4-5 hours should elapse between meals of different character.

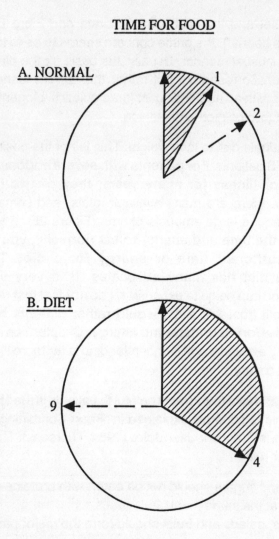

TIME FOR FOOD

A. NORMAL

B. DIET

Figure 25   Time for food

The normal individual usually spends between 1-2 hours per day preparing and consuming food. For those on diets, this time is greatly increased to 4 hours and can be as much as 9 hours. Before starting a diet, the time required should be carefully calculated.

How does the Hay System work in PVFS patients? Complete answers are not available. However, in patients with severe abdominal complaints or long illness, it is likely that the gastrointestinal tract is affected with disease. **The Hay System reduces the workload for a patient with gastrointestinal dysfunction.** Whereas an unaffected gastrointestinal tract can easily cope with whatever is ingested, it makes sense to combine foods with similar digestive requirements when there is abnormal function of the gastrointestinal tract.

FOOD ALLERGIES

After a viral infection, patients may develop food allergies (British Medical Journal, 1981; 283: 1086) which can result in severe and worrying symptoms. The vast majority of PVFS patients do *not* have food allergies. **Food allergy is immediate reactions to tiny amounts of some specific foods.** It is often a life-long problem and total avoidance of the specific food is the main treatment.

1. Symptoms

Food allergy can result in symptoms in any system in the body. The most characteristic features are : sweating unrelated to exercise; fatigue that is not helped by rest; swelling of different parts of the body and changes in body weight. Typically these features vary in severity over weeks and months. More unusually, specific systems of the body can be involved, such as :

a) chest : wheezing, difficulty in breathing, pains, palpitations.
b) abdomen : pain, diarrhoea, feeling "full" all of the time or after food.
c) bladder : burning, frequent urination.

d) muscular : aches, pains, burning.
e) joints : pains, difficulty moving.
f) skin : itchy rashes.
g) nervous : dizziness, headache. migraine, nasal catarrh.
h) psychological : depression, panic attacks, paranoia.

As can be seen from the extensive list above, food allergies can produce similar complaints to those of PVFS. This is not surprising as both may be caused by abnormalities in the immune system. The situation is further complicated as patients with PVFS can develop food allergies, and symptoms may be due to either. Fortunatetly, it is possible to separate the two conditions by testing for food allergies. **If symptoms are due to food allergies, they will go away when the causative food is avoided.** If symptoms are due to PVFS, they will not go away with a change of diet. Instead, only the slow recovery from the viral infection will see the disappearance of the complaints.

2. Tests

Testing for food allergy can be done in a number of ways either in hospital or at home. In both instances, it is important that the patients should first consult their doctors to determine if there are any other causes for their complaints. **Only when no other cause can be found, should food testing start.** Best results are achieved when testing is done with the approval and cooperation of the patient's doctor. In patients with an underlying disease (apart from PVFS), or those who are on drugs or tablets, it is mandatory that the patient's doctor knows of the patient's intention to test himself for a food allergy.

The simplest method of testing is the exclusion diet. Over a period of weeks, various foods or groups of foods are introduced into the diet and their effects observed. If there is no adverse effect, the food is excluded as a possible cause of the symptom. Ideally, the patient should start with a **5-day fast,** however, as this is very difficult for working people, it is more appropriate for those being tested in hospital. **An alternative start is to eat pork (or fish) for 3 meals a day for 5 days.** During this time no other food is eaten. As much spring water (bottle Malvern water) as desired can be drunk, but tap water is avoided (because of impurities, especially chlorine).

After the 5 days, a suspected food is eaten by itself instead of the evening meal (if a drink is to be tested, it is drunk after the usual meal of pork or fish). **If the food is causing an allergy, symptoms return within a few hours.** In this way, different foods and drink are slowly incriminated or excluded. Records must be detailed and all food taken every day must be recorded. If one particular food produces a severe reaction, the testing should not stop as that patient may be allergic to more than one food or group of foods.

Severe reactions may be stopped by drinking a tablespoon of sodium bicarbonate (bicarbonate of soda) in a half-pint of warm water. The sodium bicarbonate produces diarrhoea and so gets rid of the offending food. The theory behind starting with 5-days of meat (Cave Man diet) is that man has been eating meat for thousands of years and it is thus less likely to cause allergy. Whereas, only much later did man start to eat cereals and sugars and so these are more likely to cause allergy.

Hospital testing is more complete, but unfortunately there are few of these specialised units. Patients are starved for 5-days, but during this time they can drink as much spring water as they want. **If there is no improvement after the 5 days, the patient does not have a food allergy.** Improvement in symptoms suggests food allergy and the patient is then tested with one new food a day. Foods are sequentially tested, for example : sugars; cereals and grains (including wheat, rye, barley, oats, maize and rice); milk and milk products; eggs; chocolate and processed foods. Beverages (especially instant coffee, tea and chocolate) are then tested. Alcohol (except beer and whisky in grain-sensitive individuals) and tobacco are rare causes of allergy. In hospitals, other tests such as skin tests or testing of blood for particular IgE antibodies can also be performed.

The end result of testing is that patients should know they have a food allergy. **No improvement during the 5-day fast or the 5-day diet of pork implies that there is no food allergy.** If there is a food allergy, at the end of testing the patient should have a list of foods that produce symptoms. These foods can be confirmed as a cause of problems by **"challenging".** This is the introduction of the food at a later date to see if symptoms are still produced. **Some patients find, after several months, that they are able to eat a particular food without side-effects when previously the same food produced symptoms.**

3. Tests Within Tests

Testing is not an easy matter. **Apart from time, effort and the necessity to record all foods eaten and their effects, the results may not be what they appear to be.** There may be tests within tests. Answers to tests, like answers to questions, depend on the way they are designed. This can be illustrated by the story:

Judge : "How could you swindle people who trusted in you?"
Accused : "But, your honour, people who do not trust you cannot be swindled."

The Judge should have asked : "How could you swindle people?" as this was the question that he wanted answered. People who are involved in food allergy testing must remember two things which may complicate the answers they get. The first is a condition called **"masking"** and the second is the presence of **chemicals.**

Masking is the peculiar situation that arises when eating the food that causes the allergy results in the disappearance of the symptoms. It is similar to alcoholics who get up in the morning feeling terrible until they have a drink, then, they feel better. With masking the patient has symptoms (such as headache or catarrh) which go away when he eats a particular food (for example, chocolate, eggs, coffee). **Unless he eats these foods regularly, symptoms return; but, if he does not eat the offending food for 3 days, he gets better completely.** The explanation is that the body tries to overcome the allergy (caused by the food) by injecting a substance into the bloodstream which gives the body a "boost." The body then gets used to having these "boosts," and there are withdrawal symptoms if there are no "boosts" (from eating the offending food). **These symptoms only last 3 days, after which patients return to normal and feel much better - even better than they did from their daily "boosts."**

Chemicals in food and in the environment can also produce allergy. Thus a patient may react to tinned peaches, but be able to eat fresh peaches. The process of preparing foods for a tin, and in some cases the tins themselves, can result in the patient eating chemicals without knowing it. **It may be these chemicals that the patient is reacting to rather than the food itself.** If a patient suspects that this applies to him, he should test himself with fresh foods. Chemicals present in the atmosphere may also cause allergy (Annals of Allergy,

1977; 38: 245- 51), and patients may react to paint, newsprint, household gas, pressed or wood chip boards. These reactions to "twentieth century" products are extreme and rare, but do occur.

4. Pseudo-Food Allergy

This is when the patient has an underlying psychological problem rather than a food allergy (British Medical Journal, 1986; 292: 221-2). **The patient focuses on food allergy as the solution to his problems. There is an immediate placebo benefit from the exclusion of a particular food. However, it does not last.** To maintain improvement, there has to be continual placebo benefits from continual exclusion of foods. As this continues, there can be a serious risk of malnutrition. This is another reason why patients should not undertake food allergy testing without first consulting their doctor. Early morning awakening, frequent changes in mood and disturbances in appetite and energy suggest an underlying psychological problem.

5. Alternative Foods

The important lesson from testing for food allergy is that patients need to find out as much as possible about themselves. It is not sufficient to know that there is a reaction to sugar cubes. Certainly, avoiding all sugar will prevent the recurrence of symptoms, but it will also produce unnecessary restrictions on a patient's lifestyle. Thus, a patient should explore alternative foods, for example there may not be a reaction to unrefined (brown) sugar. Similarly, there may be a reaction to cow's milk but not to goat's milk. **There are numerous alternative foods and it is worth testing most of them.** Allergy tends to occur with a food that is eaten often (if not daily), and therefore a considerable change of behaviour is required if an alternative food is not found.

6. Commercial Allergy Testing

Facilities for testing for allergies in the National Health Service are limited. This has prompted a growth area in commerical testing for allergies. A Consumer's Association "Which?" magazine survey, with the help of two London Hospitals (Lancet, 1987; i: 92-4), has **revealed many inadequacies in the commercial tests.** They found that commercial tests on hair and blood were unable to detect some allergies; and, that there was poor reproducibility, i.e. when duplicate tests were sent there were different results. A worrying finding was that the commercial tests appeared to report many non-existent allergies. The tests cost between £8.00 and £65.00. **Cytotoxic tests** are used to define masked food allergy, but unfortunately, these tests are not widely available.

IgE antibodies (RAST) tests are available in most hospitals. There is national, external quality assessment of these tests; and, if local hospitals cannot do the tests, there should be no difficulty in arranging for another hospital to test the blood.

Much harm can be done if a patient receives an incorrect result. At the moment, it seems wise to stick to the hospital IgE tests. Anyway, in food allergy, laboratory tests are secondary to the actual testing with suspected foods. Money may be better spent in testing oneself properly, rather than in the use of commercial tests that are unreliable.

FOOD INTOLERANCE

Food intolerance differs from food allergy in that with **food** intolerance large quantities of the food are required and reactions are not immediate, occurring many hours later. The usual skin tests and laboratory tests which are used to diagnose food allergy are negative with food intolerance.

Diagnosis of food intolerance depends on demonstrating symptoms with exposure to the offending food. Patients should start with an exclusion diet as in the food allergy section. Unlike food allergy, the reaction in food intolerance can be delayed and occur the next day. However, similar to food allergy if symptoms do not improve on a 5 day diet of pork or fish, food intolerance is unlikely. Food intolerance in PVFS patients is likely to be more common than food allergy. Patients who are recently ill and who do not have abdominal complaints are unlikely to have food allergy or intolerance. The vast majority of PVFS patients are better spending time to understand energy rather than dieting. The fifth step to better recovery is the understanding of food and diets and applies to only a few patients. Patients who have severe abdominal complaints or illness for many years should consider diets.

ALCOHOL

Alcohol intolerance is common in PVFS patients and may affect up to 30% of these patients. Alcohol can adversely affect patients with PVFS in at least two ways. It may be part of a food allergy, alternatively there may be direct action of the alcohol. Surprisingly, it is not excessive alcohol intake (patients with PVFS are rarely alcoholic), but moderate amounts that can have profound effects. Alcohol is a drug with a large number of actions on various tissues in the body. For healthy people, the most noticeable action is on the brain. Inhibitions are removed and can result in hyperactivity. Another effect of alcohol is the dilatation of blood vessels which result in the feeling of warmth.

For many PVFS patients, there is usually profound tiredness and exhaustion after alcohol. The reason for this is unclear. Yet, one possible explanation is that activity plus dilatation of the blood vessels results in the pooling of blood in the tissues, especially in the muscles. This causes a reduced oxygen supply to the muscles and a build-up of harmful metabolites. Although these effects will also occur in normal individuals, they would be able to recover quickly as they have normal muscle function. However, patients with PVFS have abnormal muscle function and will thus take longer to recover. **The effect will be similar to that of excessive exercise, prolonged tiredness and fatigue.**

Patients may complain of a variety of symptoms after an alcoholic drink. The diary is the best way of showing a relationship between alcohol and symptoms. If patients find that they suffer after a drink, they should identify the drink. The quantity of alcohol differs in various drinks, so a patient reacting purely to alcohol may find that beer has less of an effect as compared to spirits. Another feature of different alcoholic beverages are the impurities that may be present. Thus, a patient may have debilitating catarrh after red wine, but may be tolerant to white wine. **As with food allergies, it is worth determining precisely what effects are produced by particular drinks.** Unfortunately, many patients may find it easier to avoid alcohol. Like Noah, the first man to discover alcohol (Genesis, 9, 21), patients with PVFS should beware of its effects.

WHAT TO DO?

To ask someone to test himself for food allergy is to ask

a lot. It is like asking someone to run a marathon. There is a lot of work involved over a long time. This is the fifth step to better recovery, and fortunately, it only applies to a few patients. **It is best left until patients know more about themselves, at least after spending six months on the first four steps of better recovery (Chapters Seven to Eleven).**

After six months of keeping a diary, there can be careful consideration of food testing if there has been no improvement. **It is worth discussing the matter with your doctor, and asking him to test for blood IgE antibodies to common food allergens.** This is a simple blood test and may indicate that there is an allergy. While this is being done, the patient should consult his diary and see, if over the six months, there has been any noticeable adverse effect of particular foods. Another useful exercise is to read a few books on allergy and the difficulty in testing for allergens.

The best results are when the diary, or the IgE antibodies indicate a probable allergy. Such patients may then feel sufficiently motivated to start testing. **Food testing is very demanding; it is better not to attempt it, if it is unlikely to be done properly.** In patients with PVFS, symptoms in the majority are related to poor understanding of energy.

SUMMARY

1. Patients with PVFS require a healthy diet as food is required for healing the body.

2. The fifth step to better recovery is an understanding of food and diets. This step does not apply to most patients, but only to patients with severe abdominal complaints or illness for many years.

3. The diet that is the most useful is the Hay System and this can be adopted before food testing. This diet reduces the workload in an individual with gastro intestinal dysfunction.

4. Testing for food allergies or intolerance can be done in hospital or at home. Before starting such tests, patients should see their doctor. Carefully consider if you have the time and energy to test for allergies.

5. Patients do not have a food allergy or intolerance if they are not better after 5 days of fasting or 5 days of a pork (or fish) diet.

6. If they are better after a 5-day fast, foods or groups of foods are introduced (one food a day) into the diet. In this way foods are either incriminated or excluded as a cause of the allergy.

7. Sodium bicarbonate in warm water can stop an allergic reaction.

8. Two complicating factors ('tests within tests') in food testing are 'masking' and chemicals in food and the environment.

9. Many patients suffer adverse effects from small amounts of alcohol. In a few, it is due to an allergy. In most, prolonged tiredness and fatigue may be a result of other effects of alcohol. These effects may only occur with some alcoholic drinks.

10. Patients should not consider testing until at least six months have been spent on the first four steps to better recovery. Most patients do not have a food allergy or intolerance.

CHAPTER THIRTEEN
MANAGEMENT

Sir Edward Halse, physician to King George III, was amazed at the success of a quack doctor called Dr Rock. When these two gentlemen first met, he could not resist asking :

"How can you, without any education, skill or knowledge of medicine live in such style with a town house, country house and carriage? Whereas I, allowed to posses some knowledge have none of these things."

Rock, slightly amused, replied : "How many people have passed since you asked your question?"

"About a hundred" answered the doctor.

"And how many out of that hundred think you possess common sense?"

"Possibly one" replied Sir Edward.

"Then", said Rock "That one comes to you, and I take care of the other ninety-nine."

Patients with (PVFS) are less than one in a hundred, nevertheless, **it is equally important for these patients to be discerning.** There are many who feel able to give advice, and indeed the problem for patients with PVFS is that they are often given too much advice. Yet, patients need help. Ideally, their doctor should be aware of their illness, its natural history and the value of supportive treatment. **Equally, patients should understand their affliction and have realistic expectations of their doctors and themselves.**

DIAGNOSIS

The diagnosis of PVFS has been discussed in Chapter Five. **It is a clinical diagnosis and there are no specific laboratory tests.** It is also what is called a "diagnosis of exclusion" (ie other conditions which may produce similar symptoms have to be excluded), and so the diagnosis is best made by a doctor. **In the vast majority of patients, there is no evidence of a continuing viral infection.** In a small number, there is evidence such as IgM antibodies (especially to Coxsackie or Epstein-Barr viruses), or raised IgG antibody titres. Many patients may have raised IgG antibody to measles virus, but this is probably a reflection of disturbed immune function rather than continuing infection. It is rare to grow the causative virus in samples from the patient.

Other presumptive evidence that may be found in PVFS are low IgA levels, circulating immune complexes, changes in T (helper), T (suppressor) and natural killer cells (Chapter Four). **It must be emphasised that completely normal results are very common in patients with PVFS.** Although abnormal results can be comforting, both for patient and doctor, they are *not* necessary to make the diagnosis.

Many patients are dismayed at the time taken for doctors to make the diagnosis. This caution of doctors is frequent when the diagnosis is one of exclusion. In the past, in one study, the diagnosis was made only when 92% were ill for more than one

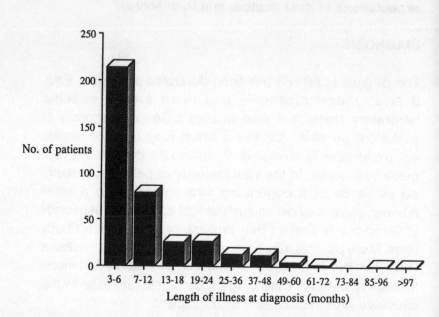

Figure 26   Length of illness at diagnosis

In a recent study, diagnosis of the illness has greatly improved. The majority of patients (56%) were diagnosed when they were ill for 3-6 months, and only 9% were ill for more than 2 years.

(Ho-Yen DO, Scottish Medical Journal, 1988; 33 : 368-9)

year and 39% were ill for more than 11 years. **Matters are now greatly improved and the majority of patients are diagnosed within 6 months (Figure 26).**

MEDICAL MANAGEMENT

There is no specific treatment for PVFS, but supportive help can be of great value. The word "supportive" in this context is used to mean treatment that can be given to patients to alleviate their symptoms, but without affecting the main illness. Patients with PVFS have a chronic illness, and therefore visit their doctor much more often than other individuals of the same age. The mental attitude of the doctor to these patients is crucial. The following are most important :

1. Accept PVFS As the Diagnosis

This is primarily a diagnosis of exclusion, and therefore other causes of the patient's symptoms must be considered (Chapter Five). **A strong point in favour of the diagnosis is the typical history of a previously healthy, athletic individual who has delayed recovery from a viral illness.** An attempt should be made to establish if there is continuing infection by taking appropriate blood and other samples. In most cases the results will be negative, but they are also useful in establishing a baseline in a group of patients with many problems. Immunological studies, especially assessing T (helper), T (suppressor) and natural killer cells, may add further weight to the diagnosis (Chapter Four).

2. Identify the Patients' Problems

As with most individuals accustomed to good health, patients with PVFS do not adjust well to being ill. Their complaints are many. Their anger and frustration with the medical profession and their situation is intense. Time has to be spent in penetrating this barrier of anger and frustration. In many, the principal complaint is fatigue. For others, it may be specific (for example, pain in the muscles, dizziness). **Other causes of specific complaints have to be excluded and generally these are more amenable to symptomatic relief, and help to establish a good relationship between patient and doctor.**

3. Encourage Patients To Help Themselves

Initially, patients spend a lot of time talking about their illness to anyone who is prepared to listen. At this stage, the patients expect the medical profession to produce a dramatic cure. After some months or years, patients enter the next stage in which they stop talking about the illness, and turn to fringe medicine for a cure. This progression in the patient's behaviour and attitude is a reflection of the limitations of currently available medical treatment. **Often, too, doctors may not be aware that the patient's confidence in them is at a low level.**

The answer is to encourage patients to help themselves. **The change from finding one's own solutions to problems, rather than expecting someone else to do so is a major one.** It is the start of better recovery. Briefly, the approach that is advocated is for the doctor to allow patients to (Figure 27) :

a) **Remain sane** (Chapter Seven) by reassuring them that they are ill and encourage them to help themselves
b) **Acquire knowledge** (Chapter Eight). Knowledge of the disease will allow patients not to expect cures, but rather, that better recovery is by a change in lifestyle
c) **Keep a daily diary** (Chapter Nine). For the patient, keeping a diary is both reassuring and instructive about the nature of

STEPS TO RECOVERY

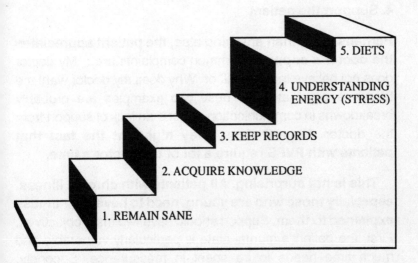

5. DIETS

4. UNDERSTANDING ENERGY (STRESS)

3. KEEP RECORDS

2. ACQUIRE KNOWLEDGE

1. REMAIN SANE

Figure 27   Steps to recovery
There are five main steps to recovery and each step is of varying difficulty. The deepest and most difficult step is understanding energy. Each step is further explained by separate chapters in this book, and understanding energy is explained in two chapters.

the illness

d) Understand energy (Chapters Ten and Eleven). This is the most important and difficult task, yet, it is the key to better recovery.

e) Understand food and diets (Chapter Twelve). This applies to only a few patients, especially those with abdominal complaints and illness of many years when other measures have limited success.

4. Support the patient

Perhaps more than anything else, the patient appreciates the doctor's support. Common complaints are : "My doctor does not believe that I am ill" or "Why does my doctor want me to see a psychiatrist?" These two examples are probably breakdowns in communication rather than lack of support from the doctor. **Nevertheless, they highlight the fact that patients with PVFS require a lot of the doctor's time.**

This is not surprising. All patients with chronic illness, especially those who are young, need to have their illness explained to them. Support should have two main objectives. First, the patient's mental state is particularly vulnerable and much time needs to be spent in reassurance. Secondly, patients require symptomatic treatment for many complaints It is in this area that the relationship between doctor and patient is tested. **The doctor has to ascertain if this is a new problem and if it is part of PVFS or due to some other cause.** As patients with PVFS have a disordered immune system, they are vulnerable to infections and take longer to recover from them.

Patients with many problems (the elderly, the immunocompromised and those with chronic illness) are difficult to manage. They test the skill and art of the medical practitioner. It is essential that there is a good relationship between the doctor and the patient. Both need to be able to trust each other. **Where such trust exists, it is easier for the doctor to identify the patient's problems, ascertain the most likely cause and prescribe the most appropriate treatment.** The important decision as to whether a symptom is due to PVFS, or to something else is for the doctor to make.

KNOWLEDGE OF PVFS

Medical knowlege of PVFS is in its infancy. This is not because the syndrome is new. Indeed, there are extensive descriptions of the disorder, probably at least as early as the seventeenth century (Chapter Three). However, it is only recently that there has been a comparative explosion of knowledge and understanding of PVFS. This change has been due to a combination of social circumstances and medical education. **In the past, medical students were taught that recovery from viral illnesses occurs within weeks.** If the patient did not recover, it was because of "low moral fibre" or even "malingering". As with many other dogma, there are exceptions. PVFS is one exception to quick recovery from viral illness.

Social circumstances have also changed in this time. **In particular, individuals have greater expectation of the medical profession and society spends more time and effort on being well.** These latter two factors have combined to motivate patients with PVFS to keep seeing their doctor. Much of the recent research into PVFS has been prompted by patients insisting that they are ill, and eventually the doctor finding evidence to support their claims. In some cases, the doctors themselves have been ill and faced with scepticism, they have instigated their own research. **Thus, a combination**

of factors has contrived to increase research and interest in PVFS. In retrospect, it is not surprising that an illness which produces such morbidity should eventually force itself to the attention of the medical profession.

Current medical knowledge allows some definite statements to be made about PVFS. The most important is that the disease exists. To most sufferers, this may appear to be an obvious statement, yet, until recently many medical practitioners did not accept the existence of the illness. For medical progress to be made, the first major step is the general acceptance of the disease entity. Only then can there be widespread cooperation, observation, research and funding into the condition. This stage has been reached and now there is every likelihood of major breakthroughs in our understanding of PVFS. **A critical question is what causes the disease.** The answer to this question is not easy and there is likely to be a number of factors. At the moment, it appears that the most important mechanism is immunological. In these patients, the attempt by the body to deal with the initial infection results in serious damage to the immune system. Cells and organs throughout the body are caught up in the process. **It is comparable to a civil war in which innocent bystanders become involved, and the effects of the war influence subsequent generations.**

Thus, in some patients there is widespread damage to the body during the initial assault, and this damage takes years to repair. In other patients, there may not be such widespread damage, but instead the immune system is decimated. This is comparable to the state of the army after a major war. It is unable to effectively deal with other aggressors. **For these patients, the major problem is dealing with subsequent infection which may not only last longer, but**

also deplete the available resources further.

What does this information mean for the patient and the doctor? To continue my analogy of a war further, the implication is that the body slowly recovers. However, in a very small number, the onslaught may have been too much, and after a variable period of maladjustment, a cancer may develop. Such casualties are rare. For the majority there has to be a slow adjustment to changed circumstances. **If one is injured, there is little value in spending too much time in the consideration of why one became injured.** A more productive position is one that rationalises the injury and adopts a lifestyle to accommodate the new circumstances.

As medical research is at an early stage in PVFS, the reports in the literature are not of large studies but of individual patients. Observation has to be made and then its general truthfulness is tested in large groups of patients. Often, the widespread testing shows the limits of the initial observation, and identifies areas in which it may be particularly useful. The information that I am giving is thus an extrapolation of that currently available in the literature. Nevertheless, I feel that the position that I have adopted is sound and that further studies will only modify (rather than drastically change) my conclusions.

The reason for my optimism is that I am advocating a pragmatic approach. The body has been dealt a potentially mortal blow. It makes sense to change one's lifestyle so that the demands are reduced, thereby allowing the body to recover. In the future, there will be available methods that will allow manipulation of the immune system. Such methods will greatly improve the outlook of patients with PVFS.

PATIENT'S ROLE

Many patients treat PVFS like a bit of sticky tape which they keep trying to throw away. They fail and the tape keeps getting stuck to their clothing and shoes, causing great annoyance. **In fact PVFS is a giant cross which has to be carried.** It is a full time job, requiring all of the patient's resources. It cannot and should not be forgotten that if one is carrying a heavy load, loss of concentration results in a stumble, then a fall.

The medical management of PVFS requires that patients take responsiblity for their illness. Patients derive greatest help from themselves (Figure 28). Patients need to adopt a plan (Chapter Six) and undertake the steps to recovery (Figure 27). It will not be easy. In most cases it will be the most difficult task that they have ever undertook. **As with many difficulties in life, survival and good health can be great prizes.**

OTHER SUPPORTIVE TREATMENT

Many other supportive therapies have been suggested to be of use in PVFS. These are listed in Table 14, as is my opinion of their effectiveness and disadvantages.

Table 14   Supportive treatment

	Treatment	Success	Problems
1.	Pain killers	Good	Few
2.	Antidepressants	Good	Several
3.	Sleeping tablets	Very good	Several
4.	Anti-fungal measures	Fair	Many
5.	Vitamins and minerals	Poor	Many
6.	Detoxification	Poor	Great
7.	Other measures	Poor	Great

166

HELP IN PVFS

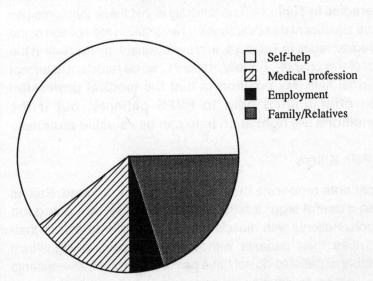

- ☐ Self-help
- ▨ Medical profession
- ■ Employment
- ▤ Family/Relatives

Figure 28   Help in PVFS
Patients obtain greatest help from themselves. Their close family or relatives
are next most important. Supportive help provided by the medical profession,
and an understanding employer can be a great asset!

The treatments in Table 14 are those that a medical practitioner may recommend. They are quite different from the supportive measures of alternative medicine (Chapter Sixteen).

As with alternative medicine, some medical practitioners are reluctant to prescribe any of the therapies in Table 14. The difficulty is that these therapies can have significant disadvantages. I have stated my opinion of the disadvantages in Table 14, and I will explain my reasons in the rest of this chapter. Equally, patients can be reluctant to accept medical help. **My position is that the medical profession can offer limited help to PVFS patients, but if the conditions are right such help can be valuable crutches.**

1. Pain Killers

If patients moderate their activity, pain is reduced. Pain is also a useful sign; it tells patients that they are doing too much. Patients with muscle pain find it easier to control their activities than patients without muscle pain. A significant number of patients do not have pain but many of these patients may go on to develop muscle pain. I believe that patients should first try to moderate their activities and understand energy. Nevertheless, I recognise that some patients may be helped by medication.

I would initially use **paracetamol.** This is the initial drug of choice. **In about a quarter of patients, sleep is severely disturbed and more potent pain-killers may be required for a short time.** Over a period of 3-6 weeks, **dihydrocodeine (DF-118) or pentazocine (Fortral)** may be useful. If these are not successful, the non-steroidal anti-inflammatory group of drugs should be considered. **Ibuprofen** is probably the most helpful. **For each patient, it is worth trying several pain killers as persistence is frequently rewarded.**

2. Antidepressants

My initial management of patients with mild depression is in Chapter Seven. **Overall, in about a quarter of patients at some time, antidepressants may be required.** As stated by **Dr David Bell** ("The disease of a thousand names", Pollard Publications, 1991), tricyclic antidepressants can make patients feel like a "zombie", but very small doses of these medications may improve symptoms. The dosage should start at the lowest possible and gradually increase until the patient feels better but does not have a hangover.

The three most useful agents are **amitriptyline (Tryptizol), doxepin (sinequam) and dothiepin (prothiaden).** Unfortunately, all tricyclic antidepressants have side-effects which may be disturbing. However, if the dose is low, side-effects are minimised and may also settle in 1-2 weeks. Other antidepressants such as **Fluoxetine (prozac)** may occasionally be useful. It is worth experimenting.

For PVFS patients, the topic of anti depressants can be very emotive. I was particularly impressed by the personal experiences of **Dr Anne MacIntyre** ("ME, Post Viral Fatigue Syndrome. How to live with it", Thorsons 1992) who **was happy to take tricyclic antidepressants at low dose to improve sleep.** She also made the important point that if you are getting better on antidepressants, you must not suddenly stop taking them. The daily dose needs to be reduced very gradually. Depression can lead to suicide and must be taken seriously.

3. Sleeping Tablets

My first approach to patients with sleeping problems is to get them to understand energy.

Many patients can be too tired or anxious to sleep and **moderating activity can result in better sleep. At the same time, I recommend relaxation exercises.** These may be combined with the traditional remedies of **honey in warm milk, hot drinking chocolate at night or a short massage.** Some patients can also benefit from a long, hot bath; however, some patients can be made considerably worse by a hot bath. If after two months, there is no improvement, sleeping tablets should be considered.

As mentioned above, some antidepressants may have a sedative effect. Indeed, a few patients have got a better sleep from tricyclic antidepressants, and I do not believe that this was because these patients were depressed. The answer is probably in the pharmacological action of these agents.

The intermediate-lasting benzodiazepines are very useful such as **temazepam, lormetazepam and triazolam.** The long-lasting preparations are not recommended. A main drawback of these drugs is that they may become addictive. However, in PVFS patients they should be used for short periods such as 1-3 weeks. **A 3-week course may break a bad sleeping cycle, even though some patients may feel worse whilst on treatment, they are often better when treatment stops.** Generally, it is worth experimenting with several preparations and it is usually possible to find one which benefits the patient.

4. Anti-Fungal Measures

The suggestion that fungal infections such as yeast infection (especially Candida) may aggravate PVFS warrants further consideration. Those who are good candidates for yeast infection are women, especially if on the contraceptive pill or on an immunosuppressant. In such patients, because of the

170

difficulty in diagnosing low-grade fungal infection, a short course of an anti- fungal drug (eg Nystatin) is indicated. **A few patients have had considerable benefit, but most are unaffected.**

Some practitioners have advocated large doses of nystatin combined with an anti-Candida diet. There are various claims for the success of this approach, but in my experience only a few patients benefit. Diets can be very time consuming and expensive (Chapter Twelve), and often the patient has to still recover from PVFS. **It is likely that candida (or other yeast) infection may make PVFS worse, but that such infection is not the cause of PVFS.** Nevertheless, some patients, especially those with long-lasting illness may have improvement of their abdominal complaints with an anti-Candida diet. I believe that patients should first try to understand energy (Chapters Ten and Eleven).

5. Vitamins and Minerals

Extra vitamins, especially large doses of vitamin C, B6 and B12 have been used in PVFS patients. My feelings about extra vitamins (Chapter Twelve) are that **they are unnecessary in an individual who is eating normally.**

Recently, it has also been suggested that extra minerals may be of benefit. In particular, weekly injections of **magnesium** have been advocated (Lancet, 1991; 337 : 757-760). Low red blood cell magnesium may result from many other conditions such as inactivity or hypothyroidism. The role of magnesium in PVFS is unproven and most other workers have not confirmed the initial results. It is probably not wise to give magnesium to patients unless they have low red blood cell magnesium and have normal kidney function.

Zinc is an essential mineral for good health. It also has anti-viral effects and is important in immune function, but is present in many foods and supplements are usually not necessary. Similarly, it has been suggested that **selenium** may moderate the individual's immune response to viral infections. However, there is no good evidence that selenium supplements may benefit PVFS patients.

6. Detoxification

In our world today, there are many toxic disasters such as Chernobyl or in Bhopal. Even an oil tanker disaster in Shetland may have considerable effects on humans many decades later. **Thus, it is an attractive proposal that PVFS may be due to toxins.** Farmers are happy to spread raw sewage over the land. Such material is rich in Coxsackie viruses and other infections which may be taken by the wind to infect neighbouring households. Nevertheless, there is no convincing evidence that such activities are a cause of PVFS.

Several individual toxins have been implicated in PVFS patients. **Mercury in dental amalgam** has been implicated as a cause of PVFS. Many patients have had total replacement of all mercury fillings at a cost of several thousand pounds. Most patients that have had such treatment have not benefited.

7. Other Measures

As each fortnight goes by, there is a new suggested measure that may benefit PVFS patients. Suggestions may be totally anecdotal, such as bee stings or electric shocks. Alternatively, they may have some scientific basis. For example, **Coenzyme Q10** has been advocated. This enzyme is present in mitochondria (which are the batteries of human cells) and play an important role in energy production. This substance may also neutralise harmful toxins, but there is no study showing benefit of this enzyme to many PVFS patients.

Unlike the position with bacterial infections, specific treatment with **anti-viral agents** is limited. Thus, there are anti-viral agents against some herpes viruses which are very effective such as **acyclovir (zovirax), ganciclovir (cymevene) and azidothymidine (retrovir).** None of these agents have been shown to have any proven benefits for PVFS patients. In the future, when there are more anti-viral agents there may be role for specific treatment.

There are considerable risks to patients in adopting unproven remedies. **Many patients have been made considerably worse, and many have been made financially bankrupt.** I believe that it is better for patients to understand energy rather than try for instant cures.

CONCLUSION

Supportive measures are useful crutches for patients. **In all cases, patients should first try to understand energy as this can help all symptoms.** However, for short periods, the medical profession can offer other support. In many cases, the best results will be achieved by trying several medical preparations. Doctors with patience and the will to try different remedies will achieve the best results. Matters will be helped if both patient and doctor can show good humour during this difficult process.

SUMMARY

1. Medical treatment is limited, but the doctor's role is critical. He has to accept the diagnosis, identify the patients'

problems, encourage them to help themselves and offer support throughout the illness.

2. The patient and doctor need to establish a strong relationship, as with any chronic illness.

3. The doctor has the difficult task of determining if a symptom is an extension of PVFS or has some other cause.

4. Medical knowledge of PVFS is in its infancy. The syndrome does exist. Using information from recent medical research, a plan can be established for patients to achieve better recovery.

5. Patients have to take responsibility for their illness, help themselves and adopt a plan for recovery.

6. There are many supportive measures that a doctor can use: pain killers, anti depressants; and sleeping tablets. These measures are useful crutches for patients, but the doctor may need to try several preparations before the best is found.

7. Many other remedies have been suggested for PVFS patients. These remain unproven; their usefulness remain to be ascertained. With such treatments, patients may be made worse or bankrupt.

8. With all supportive treatment, equally good results could be obtained by an understanding of energy which should be the first treatment. If patients find this difficult, supportive treatment can be used for a short time.

9. The value of supportive treatment will vary with each patient. It is a test of the doctor's skill to identify the most appropriate help for each individual patient.

CHAPTER FOURTEEN
EMPLOYMENT

Society puts pressure on its constituent parts to work, to be employed. Only through work by the majority can the society survive. There is an even greater pressure on individuals that only through work can you be happy. Samuel Johnson states the case : "Labour, if it were not necessary for the existence, would be indispensable for the happiness of man."

Few people realise that it is a game. There was the self-employed shop owner who was called up for jury service. When his name was called, he appeared before the judge and asked to be excused.

"I am very busy in this period before Christmas. Now, we make the profits for the whole year. Also, I only employ one person, apart from my wife, to help."

"I see", remarked the judge "You are one of those people who feel that they are indispensable."

"No, your honour", replied the shop owner "I know that my wife and shop assistant can get along without me, but I don't want them to find out."

"Excused." said the judge.

Apart from its social status, employment has great emotional effects. With work, individuals feel that they are contributing to the community. They feel useful. They are playing their part. There is a sense of belonging, income, social contacts and purpose. It is a team game and they are good to have on your team.

Suddenly, with PVFS, their role has been changed. Instead of a valuable member of the team, there is a handicapped one. Others have to do more work. The patient feels guilty. Not only is self-esteem lost, but also there is the realisation that they are helped, tolerated, even patronised. Illness is compounded by guilt and self-criticism. **Many feel that they are given a gun, and asked to do the honourable thing - shoot themselves.**

There is an excellent editorial in the British Medical Journal (1992; 305 : 972) entitled **"Without work all life goes rotten."** Its message is clear : unemployment kills, ruins health and destroys families. It is not certain how unemployment kills, but it is probably a combination of the adoption of unhealthy behaviour, poverty, stress and a poor mental attitude to life. Walter Greenwood's "Love on the dole" (Penguin, 1969) has a superb quotation :

"Nothing to do with time; nothing to spend; nothing to do tomorrow nor the day after; nothing to wear; can't get married."

It all seems hopeless. **Yet, patients should remember that it is only a game.** Life has good bits and bad bits. Illness is a bad bit. If you cannot cope with the bad bits of life, you have not learnt to play the game of life. With illness, you have to concentrate on the major game of life which is not work, but survival. **Patients must remember that to survive and get better is the ultimate test.**

Ideally, individuals should enjoy their work and their work should influence their health (Figure 29). **As this figure shows, many PVFS patients find themselves in the position where work results in a worsening of their health.** This is often because they are working inefficiently, and using a large amount of energy to achieve a mediocre result. Before they became unwell, they were able to do a job in 1 hour; with illness the same job may take 4 hours and have mistakes. **Less work (fewer hours) often results in the patient's health being improved.** The hours of work may also be more efficient and productive.

KEEPING A JOB

Most patients with PVFS would have taken only a few days off work with their initial illness. Some would have taken no time off work. Going back to work is a test of "moral fibre"; those with low moral fibre have to have sick leave. **Not only should there be an early return to work, "high achievers" make up for the time off when they return.** In this way, the patient is quickly exhausted and then the real problems begin. The diagnosis of PVFS probably should not be made until the patient has been ill for 3 months. Fatigue for 2-3 months may rarely complicate the initial illness. Using a 3-month cut-off is arbitary, but it can be useful in separating those individuals who may take longer to recover.

After 3 months of being back at work, there is a predictable scenario. The patient is falling behind at work and sleeping at home. **He is feeling unwell almost all of the time. There is difficulty concentrating. Bad decisions are being made.** He is a topic of conversation. The patient has a few days off, and then a few more. There may be diarrhoea, blamed on the "take-away", and some more days are taken off work. He has

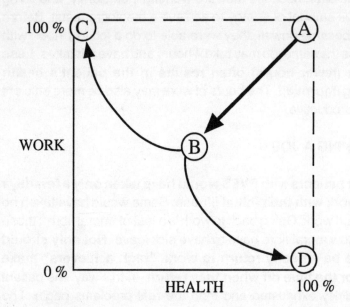

Figure 29 Work and health
At position A, full-time work has benefits on health. As work or health declines, the other is also reduced (B). From this position, some patients find that increasing work further reduces their health (C). Others may find that part-time work or unemployment allows their health to recover (D).

become a regular visitor to his doctor. There are arguments with family and friends. What can be done?

At this stage, a patient has to answer a number of crucial questions. **How important is work to me? What would I do if I became unemployed? How would I feel?** This is a time for deciding on priorities. The most common mistake is for the patient to try and do everything. It cannot be done. Accustomed to having £10.00 to spend on sweets ever day, there is now 10 pence and it has to last the whole week. **Patients cannot believe that life could have deteriorated so quickly.** There is a reluctance or an inability to see the situation objectively.

If a patient wants to remain employed, he has to be a miser with his energy. He has to :

a) stop unnecessary exertion; if the job is physical, change the job.
b) minimise all walking. Walk slowly always.
c) think before any physical activity. Use the telephone.
d) have a relaxation session or sleep at lunchtime.
e) have a relaxation session or sleep as soon as work is finished.
f) stop all social engagements.

All of the above seems excessive. It is. It has to be. A patient with PVFS who wants to keep his job is asking a lot - there is nothing left over for anything else. If he wants to do something else, he should give up the job. If all of the above is done, then there is a 95% chance of keeping the job. Most do not do all of the above. Most get away without losing their jobs. Most do not realise that all that they are doing is reducing their 95% chance to 70%, 50%, 30%, 10% .....

Less time spent on social activities can also leave the

179

brain free to concentrate on the job and home. Some have found that this coning down on the important things has produced more satisfaction at work and at home. At the start of the illness, both the brain and the muscles are easily exhausted. Brain function returns first and so it is possible to think normally after 2-3 months, provided that the patient is not too tired. **Indeed, a state where thinking compensates for activity, can produce better results.** Some have found promotion at work, purely because they use their time and energy more efficiently.

SICK LEAVE

As many patients can have a great benefit from the weekend or annual leave, **there is great optimism that a few weeks sick leave would allow them to recover.** Indeed, some patients would be willing to make a large bet that 6 weeks rest would be accompanied by full recovery. **It does not happen.** The more usual pattern is that there is some benefit for the first two weeks, less benefit in the second two weeks and then anxiety and concern because of the lack of recovery in the last two weeks.

When a patient has a score of 4 or 5 out of 10 (Chapter Nine) it is easier for a patient to stay at work than to benefit from sick leave. I believe that this is because PVFS patients are usually individuals who derive great satisfaction from work. Work is also normal, whereas it takes some time to adjust to sick leave.

If patients feel that they need to have sick leave, they should plan for at least three months. In many cases, it is 6-9 months. This is because there is great adrenaline that keeps individuals at work. When this stops, it takes the first month to adjust. There is benefit in the second month which can be consolidated in the last month. The slightly longer timescale than six weeks appears to be enough for success.

A common trap is to substitute mental or social activities for work. Patients who are not ready to return to work after six months have a major problem. This problem is usually that they have been unable to change their lifestyle. **They are unable to say "No!" to their friends and relatives, and are not in control of their lives.** They do not have an understanding of energy (Chapters Ten and Eleven).

After the first six months of full pay, the next six months of half pay are a patient's last good chance of returning to work. **Matters are now desperate, but many patients fail to recognise their situation.** Somehow there appears to be great optimism, and the failures over the previous six months are not recognised. At this stage, it is possible for patients to return to work if they seriously adopt the steps advocated in this book (Chapters Seven to Eleven).

RETURN TO WORK

Patients should not try to return to work unless they score 8 out of 10 for a month. Occasionally, 7 out of 10 is acceptable. **Many patients are made worse by returning to work too early.** The job should not be too physical. Some patients are able to start with 2-3 half-days per week and build up. This is ideal, but a lot depends on the type of job and how the patient feels.

Most patients are forced to return to half-time work. If a patient has scored 8 out of 10 for a month, this is very likely to be successful. **Patients need to think about returning to work for 1-2 months before they return.** Returning to work requires confidence. If a patient can think about the situations of work and how they may be coped with, confidence is built up. **It is not possible to suddenly decide on Friday night that you will start work on Monday morning.**

Many patients decide to return to part-time work by deciding on working 21/2 days and resting for 4 1/2 days. Although this seems acceptable, it is likely to fail. This is because in one full day it is possible to exhaust yourself so much that it takes one week to recover. As stated before (Chapter Ten), energy is obtained every day, so it is better to return to work as five half-days per week (Figure 30).

To increase your work from half-time to full-time also requires care. Usually, in the first two weeks, patients have difficulty in coping with the return to work. There is much need for relaxation and sleeping with no social life. The diary may fall to 7, with an occasional 6 out 10. After 2-3 weeks, the patient feels better and the diary scores return to 8 out of 10. **Before increasing work, scores should remain at 8 out of 10 for 1-2 weeks.**

Ideally, patients should increase working hours only every 6-8 weeks and providing that diary scores do not get worse. If scores fall to 5 out of 10, or less, hours should be reduced, as the patient is obviously not coping with work. For higher scores work can be kept at the same hours.

Work should be increased every day by one hour. Thus, patients should work their normal mornings, have their lunch break, and then work an additional hour each day. It is tempting to work a full five-hour stretch each day and miss lunch. This should be resisted as it is a common cause of patients not being able to cope.

RETURN TO WORK

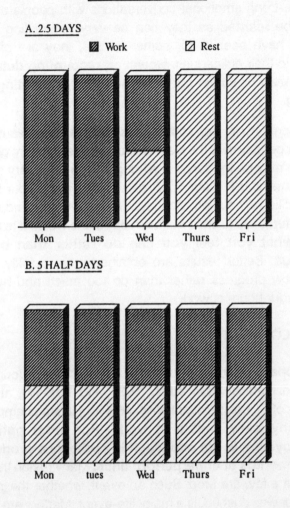

A. 2.5 DAYS

▨ Work   ▨ Rest

Mon   Tues   Wed   Thurs   Fri

B. 5 HALF DAYS

Mon   tues   Wed   Thurs   Fri

Figure 30 Return to work
It is tempting to return to part-time work by working 2 1/2 days, and resting
the rest of the week (A). However, you may exhaust yourself in one full day
so that you need a week to recover. It is better to work five half-days, either
mornings or afternoons (B). This is less likely to totally exhaust you, and you
are more likely to recover for the next day's work.

The lunch break can be used to have a relaxation session. Long emotional conversations with people at work should be resisted as they can be very exhausting. Once patients have been ill for some months, they are of great interest to their colleagues. **However, recounting details of your illness or social chat can be more exhausting than working.**

Additional hours are added on in the same way as before, one hour per day over the week. In some cases, a more gradual increase may be indicated. It all depends on the diary scores and maintaining 7-8 out of 10 before increasing your hours. One additional hour on Monday, Wednesay and Friday is a useful alternative to one hour each day of the week. **It is better to do what you feel you can do rather than be too ambitious.** Better results are obtained more quickly if you make slow progress rather than do too much and have to reduce your hours of work.

UNEMPLOYMENT

This happens. It is not uncommon. In one study (Journal of American Medical Association, 1938; 111 : 15-17), after an outbreak of St. Louis Encephalitis, 16.5% of those unemployed were "physically unable to work". **For most patients, unemployment is not sudden, it is probably a product of several months of underperformance.** Many resign through pride, but a few are fired. Such an event, whether the patient jumped or was pushed, is a major life-event. Matters are made worse, because PVFS patients were often good workers with an impressive work record. Comparable life-events can by themselves produce many of the symptoms of PVFS. The patient is on the ground and someone has put the boot in.

It is helpful to consider how this has happened. For many, it was because they tried to do too much. They exhausted themselves. Exhaustion is a powerful tool for disorientation. A person, disorientated and confused, can behave in an uncharacteristic way. They need time to recover, to think. Unemployment becomes not so much a bad card in the game, but rather that the game has ended. For a few, it is just that their illness is so severe that it is incompatible with work. For most, their own actions have produced an intolerable situation.

Unemployment can be associated with suicide, attempted suicide and excessive alcohol consumption (British Medical Journal, 1985; 291 : 1563-6). Mortality is increased among the unemployed (British Medical Journal, 1987; 294 : 86-90), but some of this may be due to greater cigarette consumption. All of this ill-health adds to the problems associated with PVFS. It is a deep, deep pit. There are two choices : either curl up in a corner, or try and claw a way out.

But what a single, great opportunity!! There is time. Time to rest and recuperate. Time to think and plan. Not many people are given such an opportunity. Horace (65-8 BC) said : "Adversity has the effect of eliciting talents which in prosperous circumstances would have lain dormant."

The first great benefit, is that the patient rests. Unfortunately, benefits do not result because a vast amount of energy is now lost on emotions. There is self-pity, often manifest by a withdrawing, a crying into the pillow, and a retreat into sleep. There is shock. Disbelief lasts weeks. In these weeks, there is greatly reduced activity. During this time the body tries to recover. Unfortunately, much energy is lost with mental activity. Emotions are up and down; there is great mourning of the loss of a job. These are common reactions for normal individuals, but everything is accentuated and made worse for PVFS patients.

Every patient needs to make the great decision to face life again. For some, this is impossible and they may not work again. For the brave, after 6-8 weeks, they attempt to find some answers. What has happened? Why did it happen? Why did I react like that? What do I want? What will make me happy? What can I get? The vast majority of the population do not have the time to consider such questions. Inscribed on the Temple of Apollo at Delphi, Greece, is a saying ascribed to the Seven Wise Men **"Know thyself"**. Patients with PVFS have this fantastic opportunity. Probably less than 5% of the population know themselves, and most who do not are dissatisfied with their job.

PVFS patients should be **honest** about their situation. **They should decide how they want to live, and if they are prepared to climb the difficult road to recovery.** The plan advocated in this book is not easy. Many are unable to change their lifestyle. Yet, I am always amazed at how much can be achieved by a willingness to learn, especially from past mistakes.

PART-TIME WORK

One feature of modern society is the greater opportunity for part-time work. **For patients happy in their job, part-time work can be an excellent solution.** It allows them more time to rest. It is positive, as the decision is made in the expectation that health will improve, and that a return to full-time work will be possible. Fortunately, patients with PVFS are often good employees, and employers are usually sympathetic to such a temporary change.

Like many other decisions for PVFS patients, it is best if patients make the decision to do part-time work before they are forced to by the illness. Sadly, many patients have financial demands which may preclude part-time work. It is often only a reasonable alternative in those families where both partners are at work. As mentioned in "Return to work", part-time work before full-time employment is recommended. It allows time for the individual to adjust to the demands of work.

For patients who have been unemployed, a new part-time job is a possibility. However, part-time jobs are very dependant on the economic circumstances of the country. They may also be very physically demanding or very stressful; such jobs must be avoided. Taking *any* job is always a weak position from which to start. It is perhaps better to only take jobs that have potential. A patient with PVFS cannot "try and see" everything. The nature of the illness is such that a patient needs to use foresight, and consider the implications of a decision.

VOLUNTARY WORK

Where patients are unable to find a suitable part-time/full-time job, they should consider voluntary work. **After a long illness, a patient's confidence is greatly reduced.** The simple routine of an every day job : getting up early, finding transport, speaking to people, being sociable, working, eating and returning home can appear to be an impossible obstacle course.

Fortunately, confidence usually quickly returns. The best jobs are those in which hours are flexible; there is little stress on the patient; the work is not physically demanding; and the patient has some control of the working conditions. **These**

requirements are easily fulfilled in much voluntary work. Obviously, a patient may need to choose a suitable job, but there is usually an acceptable selection.

If the patient starts with a few hours work per week, it can be quite dramatic how confidence is greatly increased. **With greater confidence, there is less anxiety and stress.** A cycle of benefits accrue to the patient and enjoyment in life can reach a new high.

CHANGE OF JOB

A change of a job is a feature of life today. Retraining and job mobility are not only part of the political climate, but they are a result of developments in industry. When a person changes a job, it may be either because his old job has disappeared, or that he has decided that the new job is better. The latter can be associated with greater contentment. A patient with PVFS has to try to see a change of job in a wider context : that many in the community are being forced to do so (albeit not usually for health reasons), and that he should change to a better job (a job that he can cope with is a better job!).

Nevertheless, a change of job is a major life event and is associated with great stress. It is not a decision that should be undertaken as a result of anger, or a fit of pique. Many patients loved their job before they became ill. These jobs were often difficult and demanding ones which required great energy. **With illness, patients struggle to cope, and one of the first results can be volatile emotions.** Easy irritability can result in sudden outbursts of anger, frustration and tears.

Before a change in job is contemplated it is worthwhile to properly assess the situation and its implications. Ask:

was I happy in the job before the illness? If the answer is yes, then consider if the five points recommended at the start of this chapter have been given a chance to work. If not, then do so. If yes, consider part-time work.

For patients unhappy in their work before their illness, their illness can be a good opportunity to change jobs. However, it is still important to consider what is wanted from life, what makes happiness, and what is attainable. **One must be able to cope easily with a new job.** It is unwise at this stage to have a job that is too demanding.

A change of job is very stressful because of the different environment. Patients need to establish a rapport with their new colleagues to gain goodwill. In previous jobs, patients may have been highly regarded and thus they might have received understanding. Similarly, there is little information on the new environment : Where is the toilet? How does the telephone system work? When is the tea break? Where is the canteen? Where are envelopes kept? How far is it to the wages department? The list of information can be large. **Patients have to ask for each bit of information and often feel guilty about having to disturb others.** For these reasons, a change of job has to be considered very carefully.

SOCIAL BENEFITS

Accepting social benefits is still something which many patients find difficult. There is the "stigma" attached to not working, perhaps made worse by the individual's own attitudes before the illness. Again, the lack of visible evidence of disability can make others think that the patient is work-shy or malingering. This is yet another time when the patient needs to know that he is ill, accept the consequences, and ignore those who do not understand.

Those accepting benefits and help often feel persecuted. Stories in newspapers revealing "scroungers" do not help; instead, they contribute to a general feeling that "handouts" must only go to those in need. The logic is that if there is a system with frequent checks, only those in real need will stand up to these investigations. The logic is flawed. Many of the needy, and some with PVFS, do not have the physical and mental resources to stand up to these checks.

A patient may be more exhausted by getting a benefit than not getting it. For example, a patient receiving invalidity benefit will periodically be summoned to attend a DHSS medical. Occassionally, at such a medical, the medical officer may decide that the patient is capable of work. This decision can be a great shock to patients and even convince them that society is against them. **This is not so, it is the system that is at fault.**

Many patients have struggled up many flights of stairs to attend a medical examination. To the patients this was essential as they needed to attend, and often they were reknown for their reliability before illness. Sadly, their arrival at the examination was their downfall. The medical officer would simply say :
"If you got up the flights of stairs to attend, you cannot be ill".
The fact that the patient may be in bed for a week after this event is of little consequence to the system. **When dealing with the system, patients should not do what they cannot normally do.** If patients had not climbed the stairs, they probably would have got their benefits.

The system, because of society's attitudes, works on frequent checks, double-checks, appeals and adjudications. A recommendation of being incapable of work is only the first step. Immediately, the patient's general

190

practitioner can issue a new sick note, and the whole procedure of reassessment will be started. A patient's doctor is his greatest ally. The system is generally fair and usually works well, but occasionally it does not. Understanding the system and playing the game is the secret. Self help groups are invaluable in this maze of rules and regulations :

a) **M.E. Association**, Stanhope House, High Street, Stanford-le-Hope, ESSEX SS17 OHA
Tel (0375) 642466 Fax (0375) 360256

b) **Action for M.E,** PO Box 1302, Wells, Somerset BA5 2WE Tel (0749) 670799

c) **Westcare**, 15 Queen Victoria Road, Redland, Bristol BS6 7PE   Tel (0272) 738317

There are a great many benefits available :

a) severe disablement allowance
b) disability living allowance
c) mobility allowance
d) disability working allowance
e) invalid care allowance
f) home responsibility protection
g) independent living fund
h) income support
i) family credit
j) housing benefit
k) social fund, cold weather payment, community care grant
    etc

The best explanation of the system is in **Dr Charles Shepherd**'s book, "Living with ME", Cedar, 1992.

CONCLUSION

There is a great temptation to confuse quantity with quality. Having £10.00 to spend does not mean that the purchase would be better than if there was only 10 pence to spend. Obviously, the chances are that it will be better, but if great effort is put into thinking about the situation, then a more appropriate object may be bought for 10 pence.

Some time off, or part-time work may be necessary, however, this should not be regarded as a solution to the patient's problems. **Instead, it is an opportunity to test how much can be done.** Often, with time off, a patient can become so worried and preoccupied with not improving that he does not attempt to see what he can do. Initially, it is best to look upon part-time work as "test periods" rather than "solutions".

Patients with PVFS should use their brain more than their muscles; it recovers first and it uses less energy. Because of the need to avoid wasted effort, patients have to identify their priorities. **The combination of thinking first and concentrating on the important areas of life is a winning duo.**

SUMMARY

1. Employment is an important part of life. It must be valued. Unemployment has many adverse effects, but recovery is moreimportant.

2. To remain employed, stop unnecessary exertion; minimise all walking; think before any action; adopt relaxation techniques and sleep at home; and stop all social engagements.

3. Sick leave is not an easy answer. If patients require sick leave, they should plan on at least 3 months, often it is 6-9 months. For recovery, do not substitute other activities for work.

4. Returning to work is a delicate task and requires careful planning and much thought. Ideally, part-time work is recommended with a slow increase in the hours of work, being guided by the patient's diary.

5. Although unemployment is a major life-event, it is an opportunity to consider what has happened. Also ask : What do I want? What will make me happy? What can I get?

6. Part-time work is useful for many patients when they are having difficulties with their job. It is also the recommended route for a return to work. Patients should beware of new part-time jobs and taking any job.

7. Voluntary work is frequently the ideal way of returning to the work routine with a minimum of stress and anxiety. Confidence can quickly return.

8. A change of job can be a good or bad decision. Consider carefully the implications. Take a job in which it is easy to cope.

9. Social benefits are complicated. Know the system and what is being expected of you. Get advice early and do not be naive.

10. Use sick leave or unemployment as an opportunity to identify the priority areas of life. Determine how you have arrived at your current situation. Start thinking of what should be done before rather than after the event.

CHAPTER FIFTEEN
SELF-HELP GROUPS

The young boy had been warned by his parents for weeks before that his father's boss was going to visit. On the day, he was impressed when the Rolls-Royce with chauffeur arrived. He was less impressed to see a large, fat man emerge and lumber his way up the drive. In the house, the man produced a cigar and started to smoke; at the same time, he was wiping beads of perspiration from his face. The boy stared intently. The man became annoyed and said :

"Young fellow, why are you staring at me?"

"Well," the boy replied "Dad has told me that you are a self-made man and I wanted to see what you looked like."

"Ah, yes", said the relieved guest "I am a self-made man."

The little boy was surprised at this admission and asked :

"But why did you make yourself look like that for?"

SELF-HELP GROUPS

Self-help groups, like the self-made man, may appear to the outsider as very odd, even weird. Some groups are good, others excellent; whilst some are poor and others

194

dangerous. I agree with Dr Lock (British Medical Journal 1986; 293 : 1596-1600) : "Doctors should be cautious about recommending a group unless they know the answers to a number of questions. What are the priorities? Is it primarily for patients or carers? Is its emphasis on counselling or research? Does it espouse alternative medicine?"

These questions are very important and it is very unusual for one group to appeal to all members. People are different, and the doctor has to consider if a particular group would be suitable for the patient. Groups throughout the country are also different as they respond to local needs. **Medical practitioners need to satisfy themselves that membership of a self-help group is in the best interests of the individual patient.** Some self-help groups are annoyed at suggestions that they can do harm to patients. Sadly, it is true that some patients have not benefitted from being part of a group.

The national organisations (ME Association and Action for ME) have also had turbulent times in which there has been in-fighting, animosity and bitterness. Such squabbles are perhaps a natural part of the growth and maturity of an organisation, but adversely affect medical practitioners' perception of benefits to their patients. Indeed, there are instances where the local squabbles have been far worse than the national ones. Yet, I have travelled throughout Britain and spoken to very many groups, **my firm beliefs are that self-help groups can be of great benefit to most patients.** The groups that are founded on good principles are more likely to succeed.

RESPONSIBILITY

At a time when there are budget restrictions on health, more chronic illnesses and new diseases, there is a good argument for self-help groups. In addition, there has been a loss of the natural support systems of the community, such as the church, the neighbourhood and the extended family. **Self-help groups now have an important role in health care.**

These groups should show great responsibility and commitment. They should not make their members' illness worse. The groups that do well readily accept this responsibility. The groups that are least likely to succeed are where there is no commitment. The difference between commitment/responsibility as opposed to association/interest separate success from failure.

When a group has very localised interests without overall responsibility, bizarre treatments can be recommended, some with a religous fervour. **Such groups can be dangerous to patients.** It is the reason why some medical practitioners are reluctant to recommend self-help groups to their patients. **Like much of life, groups need to earn recommendations by demonstrating responsible behaviour** (Figure 31).

One great argument for self-help groups is : one needs to be in a situation to truly understand all the implications of that situation. This is partly true and may explain why many are disappointed in their doctor. Yet, is it reasonable to ask of a doctor that he have personal experience of every disease? **Perhaps a better reason is that there is widespread ignorance of PVFS, so the group can be a source of knowledge and understanding.**

Being a sufferer is not enough. There must be a declaration of intent, a commitment, a taking of responsibility. Several groups (Alcoholics Anonymous, Gamblers Anonymous etc) start their meeting by asking new members to make a

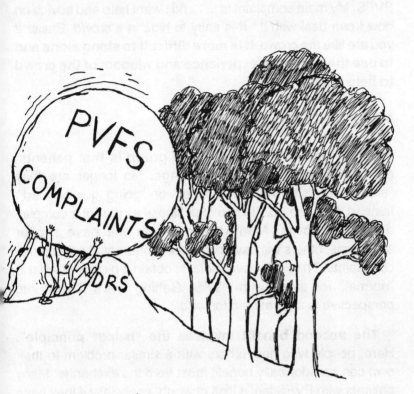

Figure 31   The balance of self-help groups
Self-help groups need to maintain a delicate balance with the medical profession. The groups must support patients and carers, but must also demonstrate responsibility and commitment.

declaration, such as "My name is ...... I am suffering from PVFS. My main complaint is ..... and I want help and advice on how I can deal with it." It is easy to hide in a crowd. Easier if you are like the crowd. **It is more difficult to stand alone and to use the collective experience and wisdom of the crowd to help you.**

MUTUAL HELP AND SUPPORT

The first benefit from being in a group is that patients' perception of their illness change. No longer are they "abnormal", "sick without a label" or "going quietly mad". Instead, they are able to see their illness as part of a complex disease process. Many around them will have similar symptoms, others will have completely different (if not bizarre) complaints. They will, nevertheless, obtain a picture of what is "normal" for those with PVFS. Getting one's illness into perspective is a great step forward.

The second benefit involves the "helper principle". Here, people who help others with a similar problem to their own can paradoxically benefit most from the exchange. Many patients with PVFS feel a loss of worth, especially if they have lost their job or friends. **Being part of a group and being able to help others often replaces the lost self-esteem.** In some groups (eg Alcoholics Anonymous) older members may "adopt" a new member, and provide a special one-to-one relationship. "A problem shared is a problem halved" may be the greatest benefit from joining a group.

The ways in which people face problems are diverse. Yet, within a group, each member may be able to see that one approach is superior to another. All are in a similar position, but some will cope better (although they may be more severely affected). **Many have found it easier to follow a friend's example rather than their doctor's instruction.** Helping each other and common activities in the group can slowly rebuild a patient's confidence. Patients who are ill often lose social skills and again, it may be easy to reacquire these in the local group meetings where the patient can feel more at home.

A group which meets regularly will soon develop many shared experiences. **It is a "bank of goodwill", with lots of episodes to laugh or cry about.** There will be adjustments or altered behaviour to accommodate certain members. This understanding and help for weaker participants can often produce many friendships. An individual going through a relapse may need to withdraw from the bank (ie get help from others); whereas, someone temporarily well may pay into the bank (ie help someone else). The approach that I believe is correct has been beautifully described as : **"You can't do it alone, but you alone can do it."**

INFORMATION

Information and knowledge about PVFS is the second step to better recovery. For the self-help group, it is important to get information to members, medical practitioners, other professionals and the general public.

Members are usually kept aware of new developments at group meetings, but a newsletter can make a valuable contribution. It is almost possible to judge a group by its newsletter. Just as national or local newspapers cater for the views and needs of their readers, so too, must a newsletter. These may contain a general article dealing with a common area of concern; a committee section, asking for volunteers etc; a diary of future events; a section of useful hints and anecdotes and lastly, a controversial letter section in which new ideas are passionately argued. A vigorous group is one in which members feel able and want to contribute to their newsletter. **Communicating information to the general public is much more complicated.** The average citizen is bombarded by too much information and advertising. Unlike the patient who has a reason to be interested in PVFS, the average citizen has an interest level near to zero. Obtaining the attention of such a person is a test of a group's ingenuity. The Breakthrough Trust has tackled this problem by bringing deaf and hearing people together, thus hoping to teach each other skills of communication and understanding. What can groups of PVFS patients do? **They will need to meet this challenge by being equally ingenious.**

The ME Association, with Dr Betty Dowsett as President, has made excellent contact with many other professionals. **Such groups of people will be grateful for up to date information, but they will resent being bombarded by too many letters.** As with dealing with all professionals, the self-help group will have to be diplomatic. Open hostility should be avoided. **Ideally, the self-help group itself becomes professional.**

General publicity, such as in the newspapers and on the radio, is an area in which it is difficult to assess the effects. **Sue Finlay's historic article on PVFS in the Observer on 1st June 1986 prompted over 9,000 requests for the fact sheet.** Most of these were from patients, or people who knew someone who was ill. Thus, the article was a great success in terms of reaching ill people, and it is not surprising that Sue Finlay formed the ME Action Campaign. Over the years, this organisation has undergone dramatic changes and is now called Action for ME and has **Clare Francis** as its President.

It is much more difficult to assess how many of the general public (including doctors) were influenced by the article. **It may well be that teaching the average citizen can only be done on a personal level.** The patient may be the best means of disseminating knowledge of PVFS.

Political pressure, aimed at government bodies or those deciding resource allocation, can be influenced much more easily. Politicians are impressed by numbers. Large numbers of people complaining, writing letters, or being vocal have a predictable effect. Yet, it is important for those with PVFS to have their illness in perspective. **Thus, objectives should be reasonable and it should be remembered that there are many other viral illnesses for which there is no treatment,** (eg viral haemorrhagic fevers, AIDS, subacute sclerosing panencephalitis etc). Worse, these diseases also have a very high mortality. For the patient, his illness is his world. However, part of recovery is being able to see one's illness as if you were well. **There are worse illnesses than PVFS; but, that is no excuse for not recognising PVFS as an illness, or for not giving patients with PVFS the support they need.**

THE COMMITTEE

The running of a self-help group requires a committee. If there is a charismatic person, things work well. **But, it is probably best when the group is so organised that there is a job for many.** Each member can make a contribution, and he/she should be encouraged to do so. A group in which 95% of the work is done by 5% of the members is weak. It is also easy to forget that the 5% are also ill and may be stretched too much. **It is best to look upon an individual member in the group as being like a leg of a centipede rather than a leg of Atlas.**

Inevitably, in any such group, the role of medical and paramedical staff is discussed. On the national bodies, these individuals may be of great value. However, in a local self-help group, I feel the role of such individuals is very limited. Medical and paramedical personnel may also exclude themselves from being office bearers, on the grounds of vested interests. Personally, I feel such individuals should not be the mainstay of a group. **Self-help groups should not be hospital look-alikes, but should be complementary with different approaches and priorities.**

A well-balanced committee will have ill as well as healthy individuals. **Those who are looking after PVFS patients (carers) will also need much support.** Unfortunately, many PVFS patients who recover want to forget their illness. These individuals may avoid their PVFS friends and not want anything to do with the self-help group. This is sad. For the recently ill, the greatest support can be obtained from speaking to those who have recovered. **Thus, recovered patients can be the most valuable assets of a group.**

OBJECTIVES

Deciding on the priorities or objectives of the group can be most difficult. My feelings on how precious time and energy of a self-help group should be spent is in Figure 32. As I have already mentioned, **mutual help and support** is the most important objective. This is followed by the group taking on **responsibility** and a willingness to provide **information** in a professional way.

Some groups feel that **research** is their reason for existing, and the Multiple Sclerosis Society for example is third in the league of spending on research. Although I accept that

202

SELF - HELP GROUPS

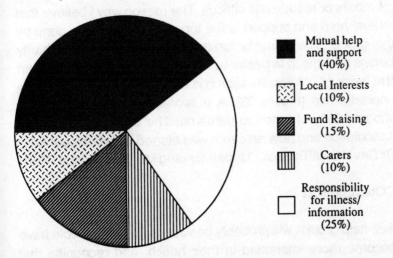

Mutual help and support (40%)

Local Interests (10%)

Fund Raising (15%)

Carers (10%)

Responsibility for illness/ information (25%)

Figure 32 Self-help groups
Self-help groups have to decide on how to spend their limited time, energy and money. Most (40%) should be spent on mutual help and support; and responsibility for the illness and information (25%) is next. Fund raising is important for the group's existence (15%), carers (10%), and local interests (10%) must also be considered.

research is important, I do not feel it should be the main objective. The amount of money that self-help groups can raise will be limited. **This hard earned money is best spent on giving immediate help and support to its members.**

Getting a balance between spending money on the group members or research is difficult. The reason why I believe that mutual help and support is the top priority is that it is done by the group. The benefits for the group are greater. Charity begins at home. **It is better to depend on oneself rather than the work of others.** Research is done by others, and is more unpredictable (Figure 33). A reasonable balance may be to allocate 25% of funds to research. The evolution of the ME Association and how research was started is well-described in Dr David Smith's book, "Understanding ME", Robinsons, 1991.

CONCLUSION

Self-help groups will probably be with us forever. People have become more interested in their health, and recognise that what happens to them is partly dependent on their behaviour. **When one takes on a responsibility for one's health, expectations become more realistic.** Self-help groups have so many advantages that they should not be seen as a temporary, stop-gap measure in the current, financial position. **They are an important, permanent, complementary adjunct to traditional medicine.** Indeed, there is even an argument that in the future, traditional medicine will play a minor, complementary role to that of self-help groups.

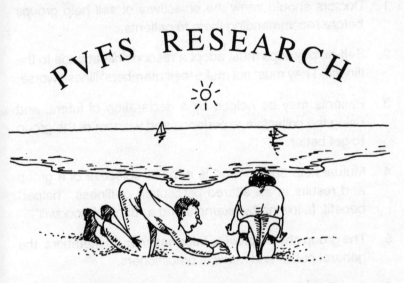

PVFS RESEARCH

Looking for contact lenses on a beach

Figure 33   PVFS research

PVFS research is like looking for contact lenses on the beach. A lot of luck is required, and it helps if more people are looking. Sadly, there are not many researchers.

SUMMARY

1. Doctors should know the objectives of self-help groups before recommending them to patients.

2. Self-help groups must adopt a responsible attitude to the illness. They must not make their members' illness worse.

3. Patients may be helped by a declaration of intent, and using the collective experience and wisdom of the group to get better.

4. Mutual help and support is a major objective of a group and results in an altered perception of illness, "helper" benefit, following by example and a "bank of goodwill".

5. The group should provide information to its members, the general public and medical practitioners.

6. A committee is usually necessary and many members should be involved in the organisation of the group. Each group should decide on clear objectives for spending time, energy and money.

7. Fund-raising should be primarily for the benefit of the group. Money collected for research must not be the main function of the group, although about 25% of the group's funds can be given to research.

CHAPTER SIXTEEN
ALTERNATIVE MEDICINE

In Cambridge, there once lived a haulage contractor called Thomas Hobson (1544-1631). His company was nationally known and his stables had the largest stock of horses. Mr Hobson cared greatly for his horses. If a horse worked one day, it was given the next day as a rest day.

To ensure that his horses were properly looked after, he devised a complicated system of rotation. However, the system worked very simply. When someone wanted to hire a horse, they always got the horse nearest the door. This behaviour of Hobson made such an impact that his name has been incorporated into the English language. "Hobson's choice" is a choice in which one has no alternative.

It is sad that Thomas Hobson should be remembered for how his system worked, rather than for his care of horses. Traditional medicine can sometimes suffer in this way. **It can be forgotten that the system in which traditional medicine operates was designed to protect the patient from charlatans and quacks.** I use "traditional medicine" to reflect medicine as approved by the General Medical Council and taught in medical schools in Britain.

HISTORY

There is also the misconception that alternative medicine is new. In fact, an alternative practice such as acupuncture has been in existence for 2000 years. **Thus, much of traditional medicine is comparatively new.** Perhaps because of its long history, alternative medicine practices are better at explaining illness to the lay public : "imbalance of energy", "presence of toxins", "natural remedies" etc. **The public appreciates the time which alternative medical practitioners take to explain their treatment.** This can be quite refreshing compared to the more paternalistic attitudes of traditional medicine.

Whenever there has been groups of people, there has always been a need to have an alternative. The alternatives that I shall discuss in this chapter have been selected. They are treatments which offer a different approach to the patient's problems, and which some have found helpful. This is an area of "fringe" medicine. **There are few objective comparisons of the treatment with established medical practice.**

Many are outside the National Health Service and so patients have to pay. **It is believed that patients who pay are more appreciative.** Unfortunately, some treatments can be very expensive. There are sad stories of PVFS patients who have taken out second mortgages on their homes to pay for treatment. Some patients have been made bankrupt. **Patients should not have unrealistic expectations of treatment.** It is totally understandable that patients want to get better, but paying for treatment does not guarantee recovery. **Patients should not pay what they cannot afford.**

I receive new treatments for PVFS patients every few weeks. Nearly all of these treatments are not tested and will benefit less than 0-5% of patients; they cannot be recommended. The more popular alternative treatments are listed in Table 15. My personal perceptions of the usefulness of these remedies are also stated. **Some of these treatments have been tried on many patients and may have a place in patient management.** However, I do not believe that their role should be major, but rather to augment the understanding of energy (Chapters Ten and Eleven).

Table 15   Alternative Treatments

Treatment	Important Action	Results
Homeopathy	Complex	Good
Acupuncture	Complex	Good
Aromatherapy	Relaxation	Good
Massage	"	Good
Meditation	"	Good
Hypnosis	"	Good
Herbalism	Diet supplements	Poor
Folk Medicine	" "	Poor
Royal Jelly	" "	See Ch.12
Probiotics	" "	Poor
Vitamins	" "	See Ch.12
Minerals	" "	See Ch.12
Dental amalgam	Toxins	Poor
Detoxification	"	Poor
Spiritual healing	Religious	Variable

Treatments may be classified according to their important actions (Table 15). Homeopathy and acupuncture are complex and will be explained in greater detail. Relaxation techniques also have good results, but dietary supplements and toxins have generally poor results. Alternative medicine often has success rates of 0-20%; whereas with agents such as antibiotics, the success rate can be more than 90%. **A lower success rate can mean that a patient may never find success.** In addition, many treatments improve rather than cure patients.

HOMEOPATHY

This is derived from two Greek words, "homois" and "pathos", meaning "similar" and "suffering". A homeopathic remedy is one that is able to produce symptoms in a healthy person which are similar to those in the patient. **The treatment causes a stimulation of body defences in patients, and these bring about a recovery.** Much of the initial concepts and knowledge of homeopathy were recorded by a German doctor, called Samuel Hahnemann (1755-1843). Homeopathic treatment is available within the National Health Service and there is a Faculty of Homeopathy, recognised by an Act of Parliament.

Dr Hahnemann was an exceptional man. His intelligence and application at school was such that his teachers did not charge him any fees. When he left school, he spoke eight languages. At the time, many of the medical treatments (eg prolonged bleeding of patients, the use of leeches) did much harm. **Dr Hahnemann was very vocal in his opposition to many of these practices.** This was very brave and demonstrates that he was a clear thinker with firm principles.

He concentrated more on studying the patient, and on detailed scientific observation. **He developed three separate approaches to treating an illness :**

a) identify and remove the cause (eg poor hygiene).
b) the use of "opposites" **(allopathy)** such as purgatives for

constipation. These remedies were not so useful in chronic illnesses, and were best where there was a single symptom. These are of limited value in PVFS.

c) the use of similar remedies **(homeopathy)**.

The method of preparation of homeopathic medicine is important. It allows the enhancement of the active component in the medicine, even though it is being diluted. Because there is no apparent dilution effect, the word "potency" is used. Preparations are at least diluted 1:10. At 24 times dilution, there should be no molecules of the original substance, yet these "potencies" have an effect. There is no explanation of this observation.

When a patient with PVFS visits a homeopathic doctor, he will be impressed by the time that the doctor spends with him. **A detailed understanding of the patient is a prerequisite of a homeopathic consultation.** Questions will be asked of the family history, the present complaint and the patient's reaction to his complaint. Further, there will be enquiries on food likes and dislikes; menstrual periods; and the emotional state. The doctor will be trying, with this information, to categorise the patient and decide on the best remedy.

Many of the principles of homeopathy are acceptable and used in traditional medicine. It is a safe, cheap and sometimes successful treatment. So, why has homeopathy been regarded as "fringe" medicine?

Part of the answer is in Dr Hahnemann's relationship with other medical colleagues. He attacked *all* of the established medical practices. In the law courts, he lost. When Dr Hahnemann was eighty years old, he decided to run his own homeopathic hospital, it subsequently closed. Another part of the answer is in the changes in medicine. The discoveries of

Pasteur and Lister on the treatment of infections allowed a different approach. **Illnesses could be treated by killing the causative organisms. There was little place for Dr Hahnemann's treatment of the whole person.**

I believe that homeopathy has an important role in the management of some problems. Homeopathy was effective and flourished when there were many infectious diseases, and when there was no specific treatment. The situation may not be dissimilar to that with PVFS. Some patients with PVFS have had considerable relief of symptoms with homeopathic remedies. **Any approach to treatment that has lasted nearly 200 years cannot be lightly dismissed.** I believe that homeopathy can offer support to some, but not all, patients. It is an alternative for symptomatic relief. It can be adopted as an adjunct to the steps to better recovery that I have advocated in this book.

ACUPUNCTURE

Acupuncture has been in existence for over 2,000 years. Chinese medicine sees all the world as a balance between two, opposing forces (Yin and Yang). Taoism ("the way") is the means by which there is harmony between man and these forces. **Illness is a result of disharmony.** Thus, patients often saw their doctor when they were well, and paid the doctor to keep them in harmony. If they became ill, the doctor was not paid. This is quite a different attitude to those in the West.

Centuries of observation have established the acupuncture channels throughout the body. Vital energy flows through these channels. **Thus, if an organ is malfunctioning, there is a deranged flow of energy in a particular channel.** This could be corrected by acupuncture needles placed at appropriate points in the channel. One important consideration is that these points have been determined empirically (as a result of experiments); thus, they work, but no one knows exactly how they work.

The success of acupuncture in a patient depends on the skill of the acupuncturist and the complaint. In those that respond, there is usually progressive improvement and only 3-4 treatments are necessary. Best results are in those who have a benefit after the first treatment. Occasionally, there may be late improvements, 3-4 weeks after a course of treatment. **Acupuncture is most effective in pain relief.** The way acupuncture acts is unknown; it may release natural mediators (eg endorphins which are natural opiates).

It is a very safe procedure provided that the needles are properly sterilised (to prevent transmission of hepatitis B virus and HIV/AIDS virus). The usefulness in PVFS is unknown. Most benefit may be in those with pain and breathing difficulties.

TRANSCUTANEOUS ELECTRICAL NERVE TRANSMISSION

This treatment involves the placing of surface pads (electrodes) on the skin, and passing a current through them. The technique is most helpful in the control of pain, but is probably not as successful as acupuncture. Interestingly, the Romans used electric eels in a similar way to control pain.

RELAXATION TECHNIQUES

Patients gain energy through sleep and relaxation techniques (Chapter Ten). **All patients benefit from adopting a relaxation technique.** My particular favourite (EMBME) is described in my book ("Unwind" 1991, Dodona Books). **In** addition, in "Unwind", Eastern techniques (meditation, Buddhism, Taoism, Zen and Yoga) are described. The place of Western techniques (Christianity, Psychotherapy, Auto-suggestion, Hypnotherapy, Biofeedback and Visualisation) is also explained. Relaxation techniques are very highly recommended.

The difficulty for most patients is that relaxation techniques take time to learn; benefits are not felt for 2-3 months. During this period patients need to commit themselves to learning a new skill. Sadly, many patients who have been ill for years are not prepared to learn; they expect to be cured instantly.

Meditation is a component of many Eastern techniques and can include a wide range of activities. One definition is "a family of techniques which have in common a conscious attempt to focus attention in a non- analytical way and an attempt not to dwell on ruminating discursive thought". (American Journal of Psychiatry, 1982; 139 : 267-74). Relaxation exercises, aided by controlled breathing and quiet chanting, are common to most forms of meditation. The object is to get out of the "fight or flight" (ie stress) reaction of modern living. Apart from the mental peace of such a procedure, there appears to be reduced sympathetic nervous response. Blood pressure, muscle tone and skin conductance also may be lowered. Thus, the whole process is high quality rest; the muscles and the mind are given the right environment for repair of damaged tissues. It is not surprising that all patients can benefit from meditation.

DIET SUPPLEMENTS

Diet and food is an important factor in recovery from PVFS (Chapter Twelve). There is no doubt that some patients on bizarre diets (ice-cream and chips, cauliflower and sugar etc) may develop nutritional deficiencies. However, for patients who have a normal diet and are eating within a normal family, such nutritional deficiencies are rare. Indeed, the most common complaint is that patients are putting on weight as they have reduced their activity. **For these patients, no diet supplements are recommended.** Vitamins and minerals are considered in Chapter Twelve.

1. Herbalism

The use of plants in healing probably dates from man's earliest existence. Fresh rather than frozen vegetables are advised. There are many "decoctions" (prepared by boiling) which can be used for many of the complaints of PVFS patients. Certainly, many modern medicines have been derived from plants, however in PVFS it has been difficult to assess herbal remedies.

2. Folk Medicine

Chronic fatigue is considered in a book entitled "Folk Medicine" by Dr D C Jarvis, Pan Books Ltd, 1961. It recommends the use of honey, apple-cider vinegar, baked beans and sea food. A few patients may be helped, but perhaps the most important quote in the book (for patients with PVFS) is that of a former president of Dartmouth College : "I never run if I can walk; I never stand if I can sit; I never sit if I can lie down."

3. Royal Jelly

Royal jelly is the food of the Queen Bee. **It is special and for centuries it has been used to treat a variety of ailments.** Unfortunately, there are two major drawbacks. The effects are not predictable; and it can be difficult to obtain royal jelly. Some patients benefit from the fact that royal jelly can relax a patient and help sleep. Others claim a reduction in muscle pain and the ability to think more clearly. Some manufacturers have been selling "ordinary" honey as "royal jelly"; and one patient ate three different preparations of royal jelly to be sure that he was getting the real thing.

4. Probiotics

Probiotics are bacteria which are "friendly" and can replace more harmful bacteria in the colon. These bacteria are concentrated in capsules which can be taken in between meals. **The bacteria then multiply in the colon and displace other more harmful agents such as candida.** Some of these bacteria eg **Lactobacillus acidophilus,** are also in live yoghurt. They are killed in pasteurised yoghurt and so are of no use. Yoghurt is also a very easily digested food and can be recommended for PVFS patients. However, the role of probiotic capsules or powder is unproven.

TOXINS

1. Dental Amalgam Removal

Mercury is present in **dental amalgam** which is used for filling teeth. **In individuals with very many fillings, it has been suggested that removal of these fillings can be associated with a great improvement.** Unfortunately, removal of all fillings cannot be done on the National Health Service and may cost several thousand pounds. In addition, removal of the amalgam causes a large amount of mercury to be released; and such dental procedures may result in a patient having a relapse. It is very unlikely that many patients will benefit from amalgam removal, and I would not recommend it.

2. Detoxification Therapies

During the early 1990's, these treatments were very popular. **The reasoning is that the large colon becomes overloaded with toxins and the patient requires repeated enemas to remove these toxins.** Alternative names for this treatment are colonic irrigation or colonic lavage (Chapter Thirteen). A colonic therapist will insert a large volume of warm water through the anus into the large bowel, removal of the water is accompanied by faeces and toxins. A therapist can charge £50.00 per visit and this treatment can be expensive. It cannot be recommended.

SPIRITUAL (PSYCHIC) HEALING

The healing of one person by another, by a technique unknown to modern medicine, is usually part of a ritual such as "laying-on of hands". **Some healers activate the patient's own energy, whilst other healers transmit their own (or their God's) energy to the patient.** There are numerous, well-documented reports in religious and medical texts. It is not often successful. When it works, it cannot be explained (ie a miracle). It is in the realm of faith, belief and religious conviction.

CONCLUSION

One criticism of modern medicine is that it is too specialised. Doctors become expert on a particular part of the body or particular illnesses. **They appear to know more and more about less and less.** Some feel that this approach has resulted in doctors being narrow-minded, even short-sighted. **The techniques mentioned in this chapter are different. They consider the whole person, not just a symptom or a part of the body.** They are also of another time; most have

CHOOSE !!

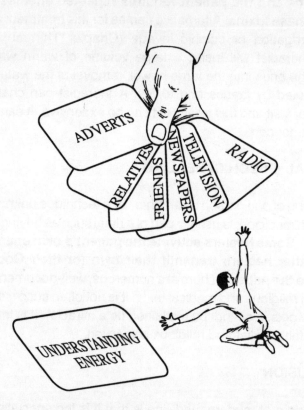

Figure 34   Choose!!

Patients are bombarded by information from adverts, relatives, friends, newspapers, television and radio. There is too much choice; there are too many cures. I believe that the most important card is not usually in the pack to choose from. The most important card, as explained in this book, is an understanding of energy. Although not as attractive as others, it is likely to be more successful.

existed for hundreds of years. In the past, specific drug therapy was not available, and there were also many infectious diseases. Successful treatment depended on understanding the whole person and using all of the body's resources to fight the illness. The position may have many similarities with that of a PVFS patient.

What should a patient do? The answer depends on the patient and the patient's dilemma is illustrated in Figure 34. Throughout this book, I have suggested that the patients should become responsible for their own health. In time, they will know more about their illness in relation to their bodies than their doctor. Similarly, as alternative medical techniques have not been fully tested (or accepted) by the medical profession, patients may easily acquire more information than their doctor.

In films of the old Wild West, there is the common situation where the hero says : "A man must do what a man must do". **The highest level of Taoism is to be in harmony with one's own nature. Thus, if a patient feels that he should try alternative medicine, then he should.** But, before he does, he should make one commitment - he should promise to be honest. If after a reasonable time (say 3-4 weeks); there is no improvement, then, he should be honest enough to admit that the treatment has not worked. He can try something else. **Trying is living, but one must always be honest in assessing the results.** As the German poet, Goethe, states : "Wisdom is only found in truth."

SUMMARY

1. There has always been a need for alternatives and the public appreciates the time alternative medical practitioners take with the patient, and to explain their

219

treatment.

2. Patients should not have unrealistic expectations and should not pay more than they can afford.

3. Alternative medicine is often "older" than traditional medicine, but the success rates are 0-20% as compared to more than 90% in traditional medicine.

4. Dr Hahnemann used three methods of treatment, including homeopathy. Many of the principles are acceptable and these treatments may be available on the National Health Service.

5. Acupuncture balances the flow of energy. Success depends on the operator, but this technique can be particularly good for pain control.

6. Relaxation techniques are a source of increased energy. These techniques can all be recommended, unfortunately they often require time for acquisition of skill.

7. For most patients no diet supplements are required, but there are a variety of such remedies on the market.

8. It has also been suggested that toxins have an important role in PVFS. Dental amalgam removal remains unproven.

9. Spiritual (psychic) healing has also been described as successful. As it can depend on faith, most patients do not benefit.

10. Patients need to choose if they should try a particular technique. There are more techniques that patients, but I feel understanding energy is the most difficult and the most successful.

CHAPTER SEVENTEEN
THE OUTLOOK

Scrooge, a local businessman, once found himself in a terrible position. He was required to travel a 4-hour plane journey to clinch a million pound deal. Unfortunately, there was not enough time for him to take a scheduled flight so he had to charter a plane. The smallest plane took two passengers and cost two thousand pounds. Determined to get good value for his money, he persuaded his wife to take her annual holiday at the same time. At take-off, Scrooge was still complaining about the cost of the flight. In desperation, the pilot said to him: "Okay, I've had enough. I don't think I could finish this journey with your constant complaints. So, Sir, I'm prepared to gamble. If you keep your mouth closed for the entire journey, I shall not charge you. However, if you open your mouth once, you pay double. Do you agree to this bet?"

Scrooge nodded his head vigorously, unable to believe his good fortune, and totally ignoring his wife's protestations. The pilot too was happy at the success of his ruse.

Three hours passed uneventfully. Then, with only an hour to go, the pilot decided to play his master card. Keeping a close eye on Scrooge, he proceeded to put the small plane through an amazing display of aerobatics. He performed loops upon loops, flew upside down, did death plunges and even let the engine cut-out. Throughout it all, Scrooge kept his mouth firmly shut. Finally they reached their destination and the pilot, resigned to losing, landed the plane. He turned to Scrooge and said :

"You are the most incredible man. No one has ever done that before. You deserve to win."

Scrooge grimaced and replied: "It wasn't easy - especially when my wife fell out!"

Although the information that has been presented suggests that patients with PVFS need to be singular in their desire to recover, this is not totally true. Most patients will recover. **There is life after PVFS. Thus, it is important that one does not lose one's sense of values.** Certainly, the change in lifestyle for many patients will be colossal, but one must still be aware that there is more to life than illness. **To be single-minded is always commendable, but knowing the limitations of this approach is wisdom.** A proportion of patients will quickly recover and adopt their previous attitudes and lifestyle; for these patients, PVFS will be just a transitory nightmare.

FUTURE MEDICAL TREATMENT

At present, medical treatment is limited, but this will soon change. **The study of many diseases (like PVFS) go through a process of evolution.** (Figure 35). Initially, the existence of the disease is questioned. Then, the acceptance of the illness is followed by numerous reports which start to document the characteristics of the disease. The illness is accepted as existing. New managment strategies are adopted, initially for symptomatic relief. From all of these pieces of

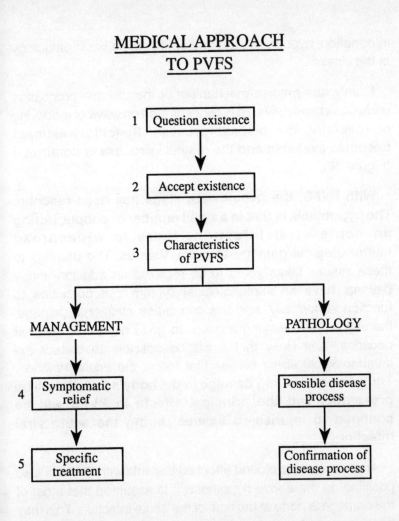

MEDICAL APPROACH
TO PVFS

1 Question existence

2 Accept existence

3 Characteristics
   of PVFS

MANAGEMENT   PATHOLOGY

4 Symptomatic   Possible disease
   relief   process

5 Specific   Confirmation of
   treatment   disease process

Figure 35 Medical approach to PVFS
The medical profession has a methodical approach to any illness. After initial
scepticism, there are particular management and pathological questions.
These are slowly answered with time and experimentation.

information, hypotheses are presented on the basic pathology of the illness.

Finally, the precise mechanism of the disease process is understood and research is concentrated on ways of modifying or reversing the disease process. **Specific treatment becomes available and the disease process is confirmed** (Figure 36).

With PVFS, the penultimate stage has been reached. The hypothesis is that in a small number of people, during an acute viral infection, there is widespread immunological damage to many tissues. The damage to these tissues takes years to be repaired. In addition, many patients have an immunological system that continues to function abnormally, and this can cause additional damage, thereby further delaying a return to good health. In the next decades, it is likely that it will be possible to correct the immunological abnormalities that follow the acute infection. **Thus, the continuing damage to the body's tissues will be prevented, and the principal effects in PVFS will be confined to injuries to tissues during the acute viral infection.**

An even more profound effect on patients with PVFS is also possible. In the above hypothesis it is assumed that most of the damage is done at the time of the acute infection. This may be incorrect. **Another suggestion is that the continuing malfunction of the immune system is responsible for the continuing disease.** Thus, the disease can be cured if the immunological abnormalities are corrected. Some evidence for this is in the single case of chronic Epstein-Barr virus infection treated with recombinant interleukin-2. Daily injections of interleukin-2 caused the disappearance of clinical symptoms in 3 weeks (Lancet, 1987; i : 154). In time, the truth will be

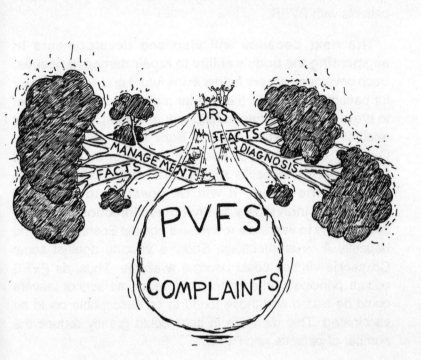

Figure 36   Effects of research
New information, facts and figures are a product of research into PVFS. The position has completely changed in the last decade, and now many more scientific articles are published on PVFS. This information will soon be used to establish better methods of diagnosis and management of patients. The boulder is rolling down the hill; the major obstacles have been surmounted.

known, but whichever hypothesis is correct, medical manipulation of the immune system will be of great help to patients with PVFS.

The next decades will also see developments in augmenting the body's ability to repair damaged tissues. Such developments are further in the future and are secondary for patients with PVFS (i.e. it is far more important to be able to prevent damage than to help with its repair). Prevention is another area in which there is likely to be great changes. Certain diseases (Coxsackie infections, infectious mononucleosis, hepatitis A) are particularly associated with PVFS. **In the future, it will be possible to vaccinate susceptible individuals against these infections.** In 1993, it is possible to vaccinate individuals against Epstein-Barr and hepatitis A virus infections. Soon, a vaccine against some Coxsackie viruses could become available. Thus, as PVFS occurs principally after the school years, all school leavers could be tested and those found to be susceptible could be vaccinated. This measure in itself could greatly reduce the number of patients with PVFS.

In summary, the future outlook for effective medical treatment is very good. It seems very likely that measures will be possible that would allow correction of the abnormalities in PVFS, and more important, protective measures (such as vaccines) will prevent many from developing the illness. Unfortunately, this offers very little comfort for the patient who now has the disease. **For PVFS patients and their medical practitioners, there is no easy option.**

THE DOCTOR'S OUTLOOK

The attitude of some doctors is to cringe as the patient enters the room. Patients can be described as "heart-sink" patients to reflect the patients' effects on the doctor. Many patients have slowly seen all of the doctors in the practice. Fortunately, this probably only reflects the helplessness that many doctors feel in dealing with this condition. **Two factors that may complicate the situation are if the patient is not believed and if he is led to expect a quick recovery.** If instead, a patient with PVFS is approached in the manner of patients with other chronic illnesses (such as multiple sclerosis), it is likely that the confidence of the patient will be maintained.

The lack of effective, curative medical treatment does not diminish the role of the medical practitioner, but rather increases its importance. The patient comes to the doctor first and he will keep coming back. Thus from the very start, the attitude of the doctor should be positive. He should look on the patient as someone who will require time, reassurance, information about his illness and supportive treatment. Doctors who have tried this approach usually find that mutual trust develops.

The greatest mistake that can be made is to underestimate the amount of time that is required. Time that the patient needs and time for the illness to resolve. Patients with PVFS feel that their entire world has collapsed. The consequent, complex, emotional problems are only frustrated by the standard ten minute consultation with their medical practitioner. Further, constant expectation of recovery next week can have an equally demoralising effect on the doctor, as it does on the patient. **The lesson may well be that the best current medical treatment is to commit much time to the patient; and to recommend an appropriate self-help group.**

The outlook is, nevertheless, very good. Most patients eventually recover. Most are young, intelligent and well-motivated. They are the sort of patient many doctors would like to have. Their illness affords a great opportunity for the doctor to get to know these patients. **Indeed, many friendships, based upon a mutual understanding and respect, have started in this way.**

As each month goes by, more facts are being acquired on PVFS. In the past, there were few scientific papers on the subject. Fortunately, this has changed and there is now a deluge of information. **The International Federation of Myalgic Encephalitis Associations (IFMEA)** collects and distributes medical information. It is quite superb (contact Ellen Goudsmit, 23 Melbourne Road, Teddington, Middlesex, TW11 9QX). **British Library Document Supply Centre**, Boston Spa, Netherby, LS23 7BQ also produces a MEDLINE search on ME/PVFS. The position is now one in which the information has to be interpreted and marshalled so that the patient can be better managed (Figure 36).

THE PATIENT'S OUTLOOK

When everything is going wrong, one tends to remember Murphy's Law which states: "If anything can go wrong, it will."

Many patients with PVFS feel that it is an accurate representation of their position. **There is an inclination to give up and to become nothing more than a vegetable.** This feeling is understandable and one can sympathise with the patient's position. However, at this stage, it may be helpful for the patient to consider Gattuso's extension of Murphy's Law. This states : "Nothing is ever so bad that it can't get worse."

The future for the patient is one in which there will be an eventual recovery. In the meantime, it is as easy to occupy the time productively as it is to be wasteful. It is a long journey and it is better to enjoy it, rather than to sit in the corner unhappy. Having read the previous pages, each patient now has the difficult decision of what do do. **The plan advocated requires the patient to be committed and well-motivated.** A lot of time is needed to learn about the disease and to keep a meticulous diary. **Most difficult of all there has to be a change in lifestyle.** This change necessitates the adoption of a different attitude. Energetic persuits have to be given up. Instead of being a participant, one has to become an observer. For some, these changes will be too much to ask, and these individuals should recall Gattuso's extension of Murphy's Law.

Dependant on a patient's personality, some things are easier to do than others. Thus, one may feel able to accept the first three steps, but not the fourth. Obviously, best recovery will be obtained if the whole plan is adopted, but if one feels only able to accept a part of the plan, then this is better than nothing. Indeed, many will feel inclined to take a step at a time. In lots of ways, this is a very sensible approach. It is reasonable to see what the first steps can do for you before you drastically change your lifestyle. **If a patient tries the first three steps for two months, he should become convinced of the value of the plan.**

The plan falls into two natural parts. The first part, the first three steps, can be the most difficult. This is usually because if a patient accepts these steps, he is also accepting the responsibility for finding some of the answers to his problems. This is a commitment that many are unwilling to undertake, and this is understandable. Some are only able to accept this responsibility when their circumstances reach a stage of frustration and anger. Put another way, when the established system is unable to provide the help that patients need, they slowly become frustrated. When this frustration is combined with anger, they should undertake to do something about their problems. **At this stage, acceptance of the first three steps does not become a daunting prospect.**

The fourth step - an appropriate understanding of energy (Chapters Ten and Eleven) is the most difficult for patients to understand and adopt. **Again, part of the reason for this is that this position is one that most of society does not accept.** Thus, society expects young people to be energetic. The need for sleep also is associated with lazy individuals. As most patients are young and often very athletic, they find it difficult to deliberately restrict their activity and sleep more. Yet, for many, this can be the most important step. **They need to recognise that they are ill, and ill people need to sleep.**

Relaxation, like sleep, is perceived as "doing nothing". This is a misconception, and relaxation is an active, complicated process which is able to generate energy. Similarly, many individuals are unable to recognise the importance of stress and relationships (Chapter Eleven). This is probably why there are so many divorces, unhappy relationships and people discontented with their jobs. **For PVFS patients, an understanding of these problems can be the difference between continued illness and recovery.** Yet, very many patients will find it too much to depart from the mainstream of society. **Many choose to be like others even though it is to their detriment. This is partly why so many have "burnt out" and have regrets.** The development of food allergies or intolerance is difficult to deal with, but this has be considered when patients continue to deteriorate despite conforming to the first four steps. In these patients, improvement can be dramatic. Further, as these individuals are the most desperate, they are likely to have the determination to test themselves properly for food allergies. **Assessing oneself for allergies** is not a weekend whim. It is probably easier to lose a stone in weight by dieting than to undertake allergy testing. Like many important decisions, it should be carefully considered and then enough time put aside to execute the testing.

A GREAT OPPORTUNITY

It is disasterous when a young, intelligent, extroverted, athletic individual becomes depressed, introverted and somnolent. Many feel that they have no reason for living. Paradoxically, few friends of patients have similar views. Indeed patients' acquaintances often have too great an admiration and expectation of patients. The reason for this is that most patients were individuals who got on with living life. However, PVFS does not mean that they should stop living, it only means that they need to change their lifestyle. **It is said that a pessimist is someone who sees disaster in every opportunity, and an optimist is someone who can see opportunity in every disaster.** Patients with PVFS need to be optimists. They need to hold on to their zest for life.

One great advantage of their condition is that patients have to spend more time in sedentary activities. This leaves a great deal of time for thinking; mental activity uses energy slower than physical activity. Many patients prior to their illness were so busy living that they had no time to consider what were their life's values, or where they were going. **Energetic activity can be the only reason for living and occupy most of the non-working hours.**

It is better when exercise is not the only recreational activity. Many sportspersons can find themselves in the position of continuing to play sports because they are good at it, rather than that the activity gives them happiness. Some exercise is necessary for everyone and for those with PVFS it has to be minimal. Instead, these patients have an opportunity to express themselves in other activities. **Many patients can find themselves in new, more enjoyable relationships with this change of lifestyle.** More important, they will have learned that in different stages of life, different patterns of living are more appropriate.

These individuals will also be much happier in the later years of life, as they will have had to come to terms with the frailty of the body early in life. Thus, the limitations of PVFS afford patients the opportunity to consider their talents and abilities, and decide on their life's objectives. Not surprisingly, many patients are much happier with themselves as individuals. This adaptation also has the advantage of preparing one for other changes in life.

SUMMARY

1. The study of many diseases (like PVFS) go through a process of evolution in which more and more information is acquired.

2. With PVFS, the very last stages have been reached and soon specific treatment and an understanding of the way the disease is caused will be available.

3. Medical practitioners must believe that patients are ill, and must not lead patients to expect a quick recovery. An underestimation of the time to recovery is the most common mistake.

4. The best current medical treatment is for the doctor to commit much time and energy to understanding the patients' problems.

5. Patients must not give up, but they should not fight the illness with activity. The illness can only be fought by knowledge, a plan and a change in lifestyle.

6. The plan suggested in this book falls into two natural parts. The first part consists of the first three steps; acceptance of these steps is a major obstacle.

7. The fourth step is understanding energy and is the most difficult. This step can be the difference between continued illness and recovery.

8. Patients need to recognise that PVFS can be a great opportunity to understand their lives, establish good relationships and prepare themselves for the later years of life.

CHAPTER EIGHTEEN
CONCLUSION

In the late eighties in London, young dealers in the city could make one million pounds for their company before lunch and earn themselves ten thousand pounds commission. They had two bottle lunches and only drank champagne. In the same place, Buddy lived. He was a teenager who had run away from home, did not have a job and lived on the streets. He was regarded as being very simple. The young dealers would pour out onto the pavement after their hundred pound lunches and stop to speak to Buddy. Buddy amused them and made then feel good. They would say :

"Buddy! What would you choose between this shiny metal fifty pence coin and an old paper ten pound note?"

Buddy would always hesitate, he would point a grubby finger at one and then at the other. His eyes would widen and he would always choose the shiny fifty pence coin. The young dealers would laugh and shake their heads in dismay at Buddy's predicament. Sometimes, a group of them would take it in turns to test Buddy. Each day he would perform at least fifty times.

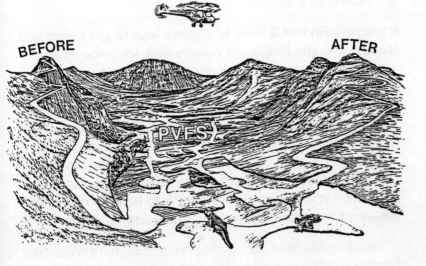

BEFORE

AFTER

PVFS

Figure 37   The bog of PVFS
Patients would like the medical profession to take them, in a helicopter, from
the mountain top before PVFS to the mountain top after PVFS. This helicopter
does not exist. Instead, patients gradually slide into the bog of PVFS. But
there can be life after PVFS. The way to recovery is there but difficult to find.

The terrible nineties came and most of the young dealers lost their jobs. One day, one dealer who had been unemployed for two years returned. He saw Buddy, felt remorse and said: "Buddy, I have to tell you the ten pound paper note is worth more than the shiny metal fifty pence coin".

"Oh yes, I know! But if I choose the ten pound note, I would not get offered the choice again. Anyway, I'm still in work and you are looking for a job."

Patients with PVFS have to choose less to get more; like Buddy, it is the long-term results that are important. Life is full of divisions : male or female; married or single; employed or unemployed; well or ill. Many patients with PVFS feel that their past was full of adventure and good times. Now, they have bad cards. They see their acquaintances, often with less ability (but more energy), doing well and apparently prospering. In comparison, a patient's lot seems to be coming to terms with constant fatigue, intermittent infections, unemployment, separation and divorce. **There seems to be only one major life-event to come - death; and, many wish it soon.**

Patients spend a lot of their time mourning their past existence. They remember times when the sun always shone, when there was frenetic activity and applause. Their current lives appear to be rainy days, pain, discomfort and sadness. **Like all mourning, the whole exercise can take six months.** Sadly, patients are as in Figure 37. They gradually find themselves in the bog of PVFS. Fortunately, there is a path through the bog. **The path is difficult and there are many opportunities for disaster.** Yet, there is also much scope for more out of life. Anyone can do well when there are unlimited resources. **The real test of ability is to succeed with very limited resources. Patients with PVFS have very, very limited resources.**

236

Are there any advantages in the patient's situation? What are the "equalizers"? There are two. First is how the patient copes with PVFS. **This is a university, an assault course, a test of survival; graduation and survival will ingrain patients with a deep knowledge of themselves.** The second is in the patient's potential for happiness. Perhaps, the only equality in the world is each individual's potential for happiness. Each person, no matter how disadvantaged, probably has the same amount of potential for happiness each day as the most privileged. **Happiness is there, it is free; but, many refuse to take their allotted portion, simply because they are ill.** Illness can give patients the understanding that they can be happy if they choose to be - every day.

Life is short. For many, it is a catalogue of lost opportunities. **Patients have to decide if PVFS is a disaster or an opportunity.** The way to better recovery involves personal commitment, hard work, self-understanding and the need for optimism. Very few are given the situation that requires acquisition of such qualities. One should remember that great pressures, over many years, are required to make a diamond - the hardest of all minerals, able to withstand much stress.

A patient with PVFS has a terrible affliction at the wrong time of life. Yet, coping with the illness and its consequences produces a very special person : one capable of coping with strife, but able to enjoy the sunshine between the storms.

INDEX